Witches & Weeds

Magical Uses for Wild Herbs

Publisher: Balthazar Pagani
Graphic Design, Pagination, and Editing: Bebung
Translation: Bianco Tangerine s.r.l. (translation: Alexa Ahern)
Editing: Phillip Gaskill

Vivida

Vivida® is a registered trademark property of White Star s.r.l.

This Ixia Press edition, first published in 2024, is a modified English translation of *Weeds & Witches: Uses, Practices, and Magical Preparations of Wild and Spontaneous Herbs*, originally published in Italian by Vivida, an imprint of White Star Publishers, Milan, in 2024.

The advice and strategies contained herein may not be suitable for every situation. The recipes and remedies are not a substitute for professional medical advice. This book is intended for general informational purposes only and does not address individual circumstances. The author and publisher are not responsible for any adverse or allergic reactions to ingredients used throughout this book. Plants and fungi that are deemed poisonous, including derivatives thereof, should not be ingested or touched in any form.

Please exercise caution when performing actions involving candles, incense, and fire.

This book is not recommended for children.

ISBN-13: 978-0-486-85256-0
ISBN-10: 0-486-85256-3

IXIA PRESS
An imprint of Dover Publications

Manufactured in China
85256301   2024
www.doverpublications.com/ixiapress

Witches
&Weeds

Magical Uses for Wild Herbs

Text by **Cecilia Lattari**

Illustrations by **Fabiana Belmonte**

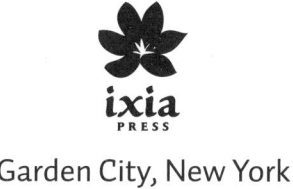

ixia
PRESS

Garden City, New York

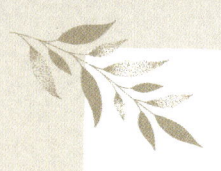

CONTENTS

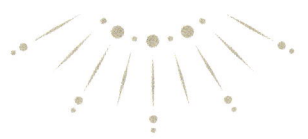

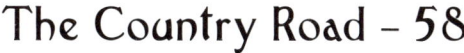

INTRODUCTION

From the window of my apartment in Bologna, where I lived while studying at theater school, I could see a small strip of land colonized by various plants. In late February, fragrant and discreet violets would appear before giving way to the exuberant dandelion in spring. In the summer, when I was packing my bags to return home to my beloved Tuscan Apennines, poppies and a few chamomile flowers, carried in on the wings of who knows what from who knows where, would greet me from that patch of wild land.

I have always loved weeds, starting with their name, a term that holds a certain magic and mystery. They are rebellious, brave, fearless. Some weeds pop up even in the middle of big city streets, straight through the cracks in the asphalt.

These plants acquire a different meaning in botany and phytotherapy books. During my college

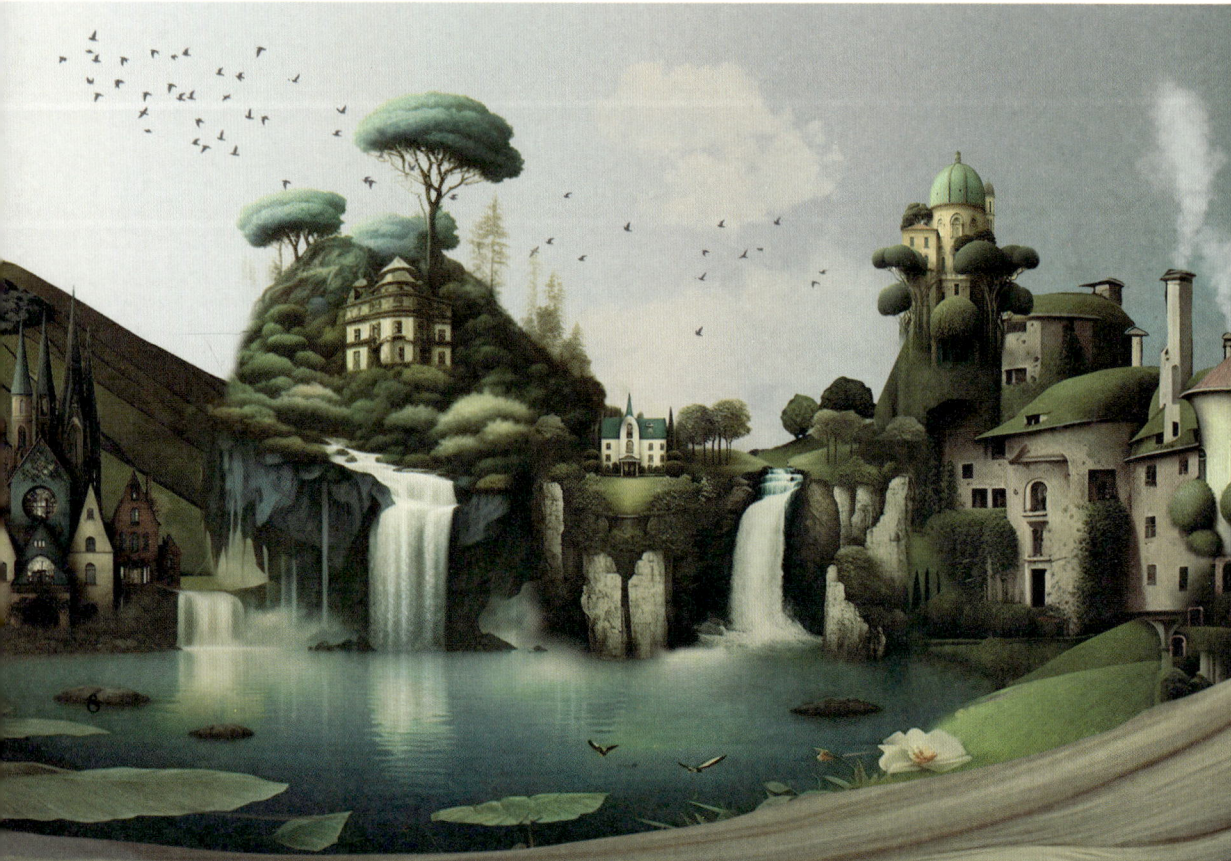

years, I discovered that even the much-feared witchgrass is a strong, tenacious, and beneficial plant, as are many other weeds.

Weeds' unconventional and wild spirit often links them to witches. They have always had a deep and intimate connection, a symbiosis that goes back to ancient times. Weeds, like witches, are often considered inappropriate and undesirable, yet they are able to grow and thrive in difficult conditions, defying convention and the established order.

Weeds are often considered invasive. They grow with full confidence in difficult places and can be pioneer plants. They offer many benefits, from healing the body to healing the soul, just like witches and healers.

The encounter between witches and weeds is an invocation to the magic, knowledge, and beauty that can be found outside of rules and conventions. It is an invitation to rediscover a connection with nature and one's inner power, to look for the beauty and mystery in everything.

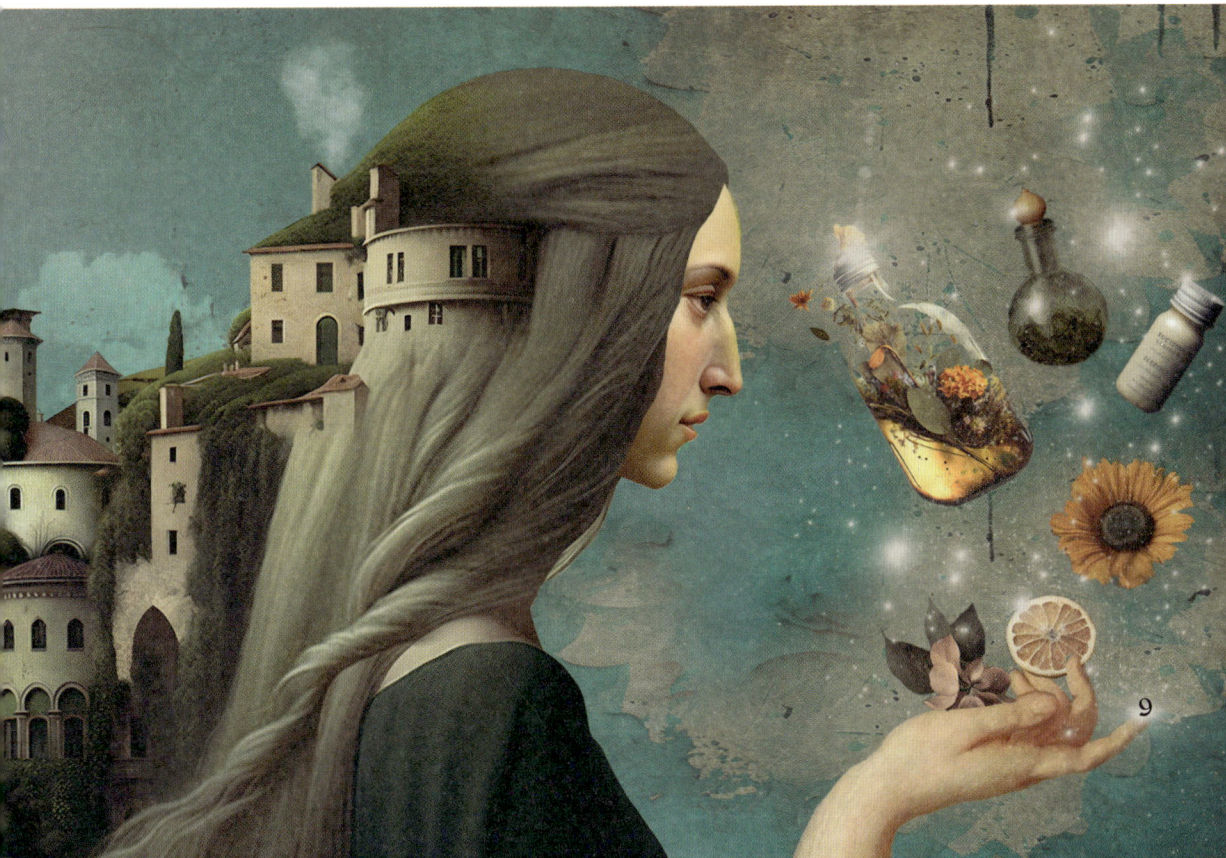

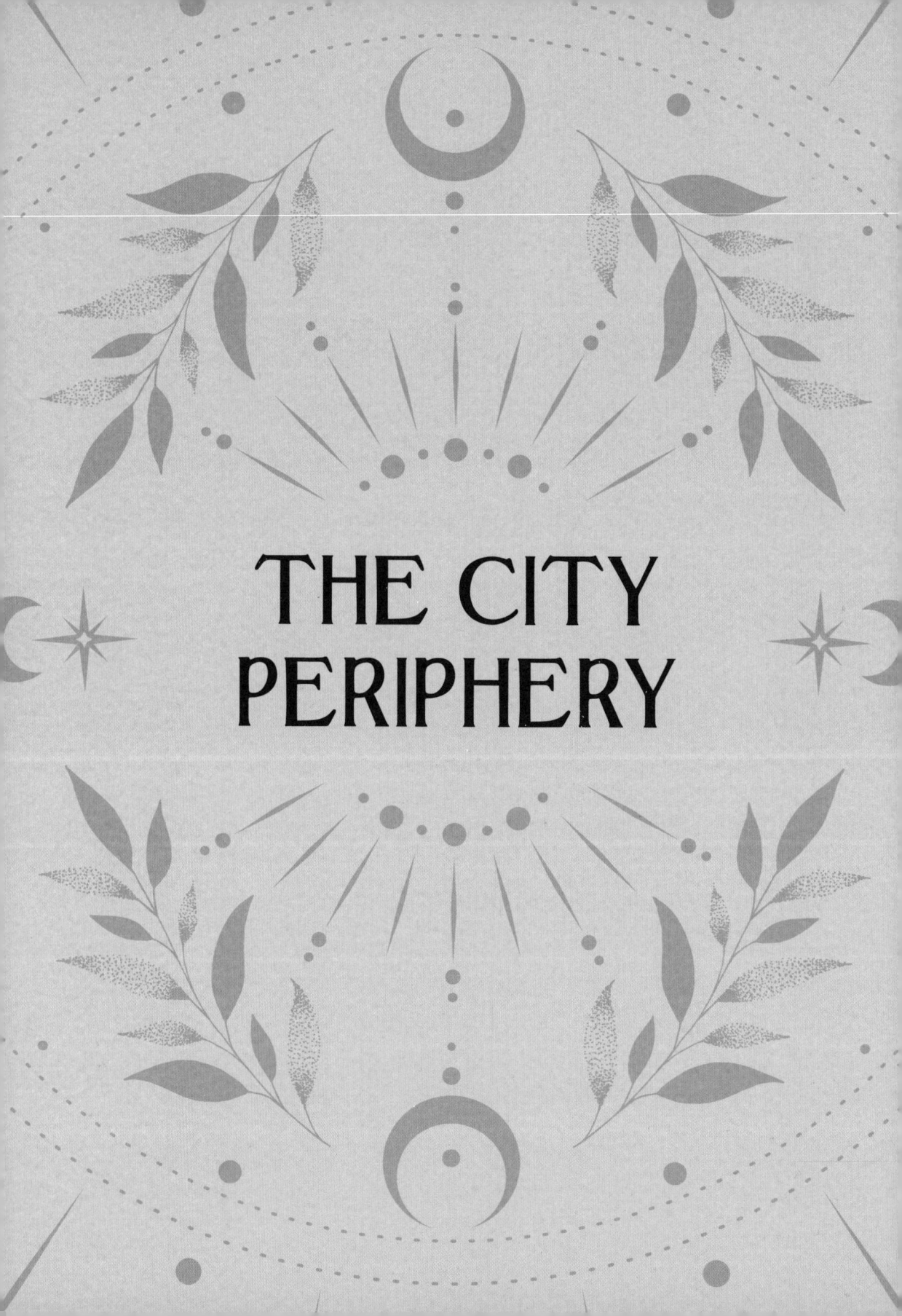

THE CITY
PERIPHERY

There are indefinable liminal borderlands where magic lives, like on the outskirts of the city. In these places, anything could be hiding a trace of magic and could transform into the key that opens a door to another world, an almost illegible writing on the wall or an abandoned magazine, read by the wind turning the pages.

Here in the suburbs, especially on sunny days, time flows differently and encounters with people are more relaxed and spontaneous. Anything can come from *"Hello! Lovely evening, isn't it?"* In your pocket, you carry some small treasures you picked up on the roadside during a walk, like a polished piece of glass or a seed that looks like a treasure chest. But only by looking down will you see the real inhabitants of these places: the weeds, wild plants that dot the landscape, fearless and brave, growing between the cracks in the little walls, like capers with their cotton candy–colored flowers, moving slowly through the evening air. The suburbs are full of magic, partly because this is where you don't expect to find it. There is a small store, on the corner of the street. It sells used items, passed down from hand to hand, from one love to another. These are full of stories, like the streets that wind from the center and reach here, the edge, from where you can see everything better. The urban witch lives in these places and knows the power of them. To those who wonder whether city witches can exist where there is no forest and no wild plants grow, the answer might be surprising. We need to open our eyes and our hearts: magic is resilient and everywhere; enchantments can be strung from sidewalk to window, from lamppost to doorstep, and on or near borders.

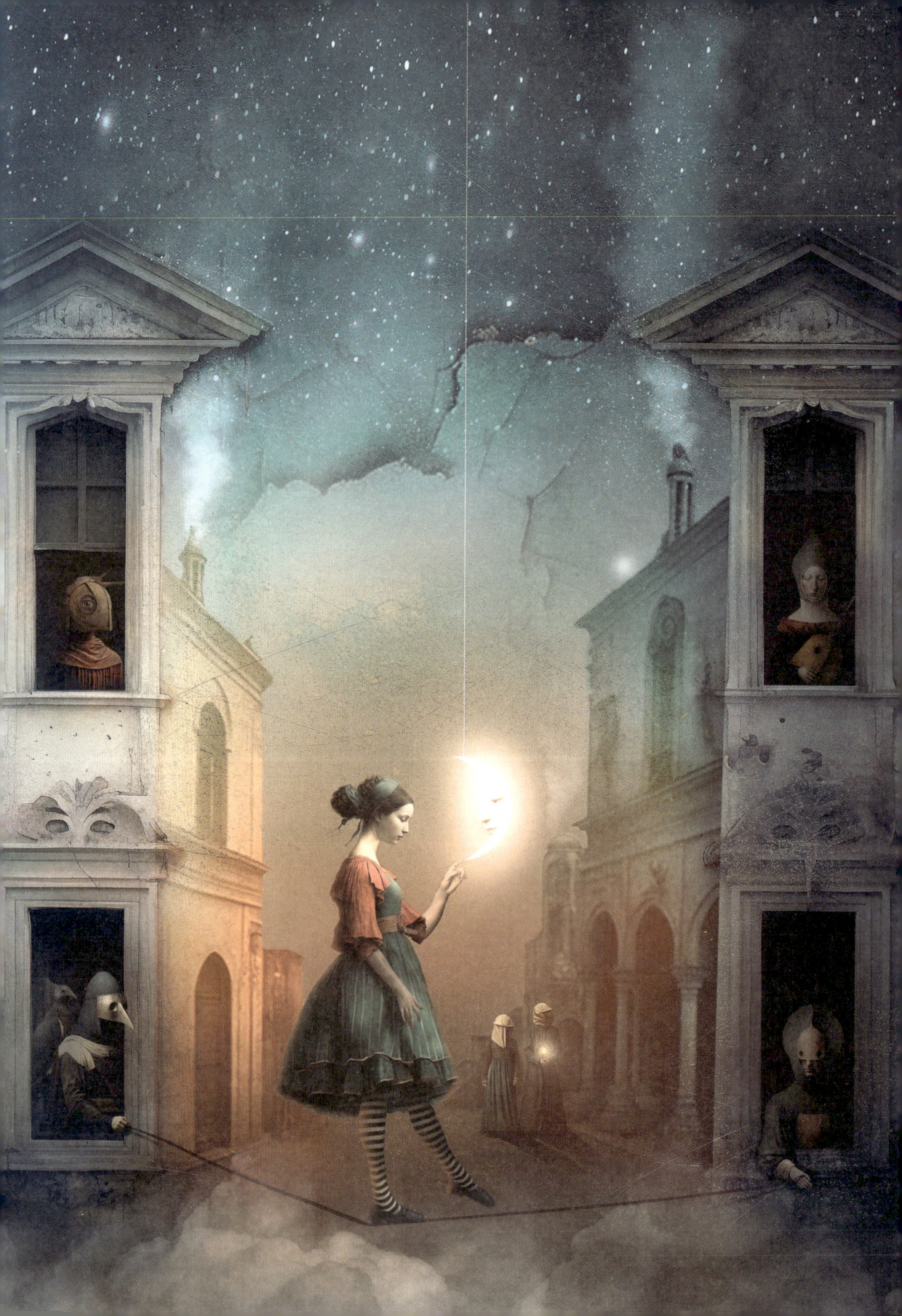

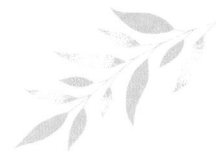

THE URBAN WITCH

—

The urban witch lives on the periphery of every city; yours is no exception. She does not need a forest to be able to collect weeds and roots: she knows nature and knows how to find it even on the asphalted streets that lead to the city center.

Magic is a state of mind, and much of it depends on how you observe your surroundings. The urban witch collects dandelions in the small park behind her house, then takes them with her to make herbal teas and infusions; she observes the flight of birds and the dance of clouds and knows how to pick up on the signs that manifest themselves in the everyday.

She is a specialist in everyday magic. Just as the whole tree is preserved in the seed, she's able to grasp the great potential that resides in small everyday things: the coffee from the coffee shop below her house, at the fruit and vegetable stand at the farmers market, in the evening stroll of two people walking their dog. The urban witch knows little enchantments that harmonize her life with the elements of nature: she hangs bells on her windows to greet the fairies, and in the evening she never fails to light a candle on the table to honor the spirits of the Fire and the Hearth.

On her balcony live her mint and rosemary plants, whose beneficial scents cheer the mind and heart. When she leaves the house, she always has a deck of tarot cards in her bag and a few stones to play with during the day, like rock crystal, aventurine, and tigereye. When, walking down the sidewalk, the magnolia from a nearby garden brushes her hair, she whispers under her breath enchantments of protection: for nature, for the day that is beginning, for the people who live in the neighborhood.

Urban witches are masters of *cledon*, which consists of being able to catch fragments of conversation between strangers, intercepted on the street, that turn out to be revelatory for us, bearing fundamental answers. But it can also manifest itself through a book that falls from our hands, opening to exactly the page that contains the words we needed to hear. This is casual magic: it happens when we are in an open, attentive, and receptive state of mind. Sometimes we need to be sensitive to the nuances of the world around us to recognize it.

> The magic of *cledon* lies in the ability to seize glimmers of meaning and direction in a seemingly random universe. We cannot control or predict when and how a *cledon* will manifest, but we can learn to be present to the signals that life sends us. It invites us to embrace the wonder hidden in the very fabric of existence.

This is one of the valuable teachings of the urban witch: *stop and listen* and, as the Hermit does with his lantern, *look for magic in the tapestry of your days.*

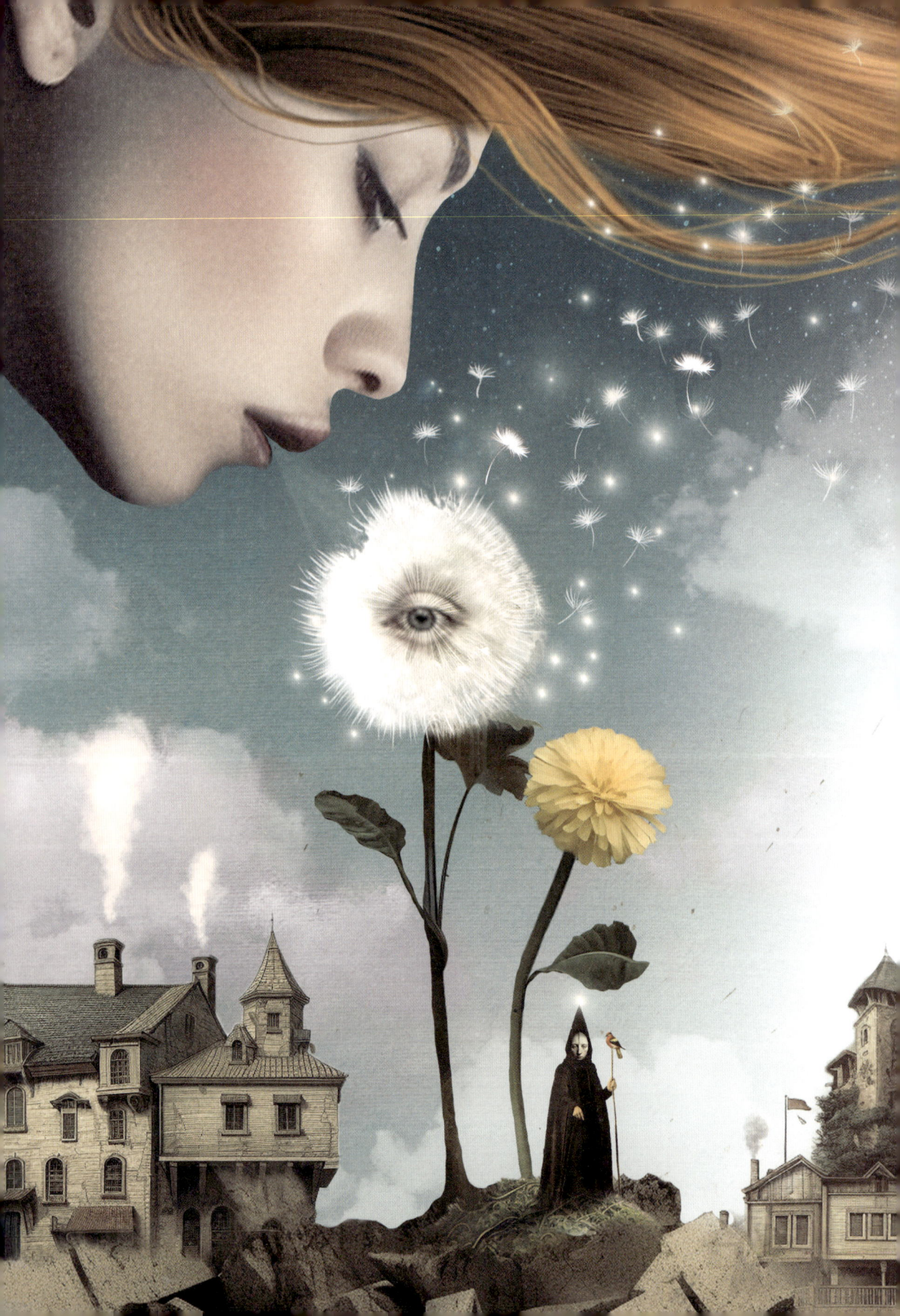

DANDELION

— Taraxacum officinale —

The dandelion is a symbol of spring. When its sun-yellow blossoms begin to sprout from cracks in asphalt in the city, it means spring has begun, and it reminds us of ourselves as children, blowing on it to make wishes come true. The dandelion is made immediately recognizable by its fruit, the pappus, composed of soft winged seeds, and its arrow-shaped leaves, grouped in a basal rosette. Young leaves, harvested before the plant flowers, are considered more tender and flavorful. The long, fleshy roots of the dandelion are also edible and are especially used for detoxifying and diuretic herbal teas. The roots can be roasted and ground to create a kind of *dandelion coffee*, which tastes similar to coffee but without the caffeine. Its ability lies in expansion. A plant linked to Jupiter, it carries its seeds far away from the mother plant and urges us to dream, bringing our gaze forward with confidence into the future.

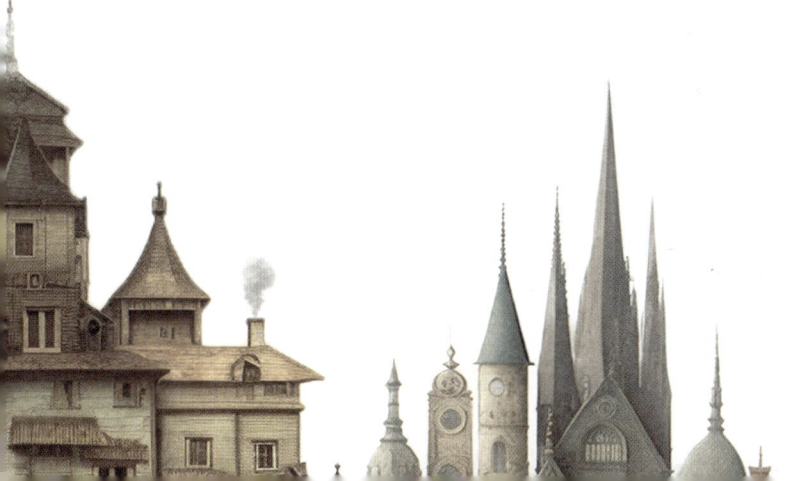

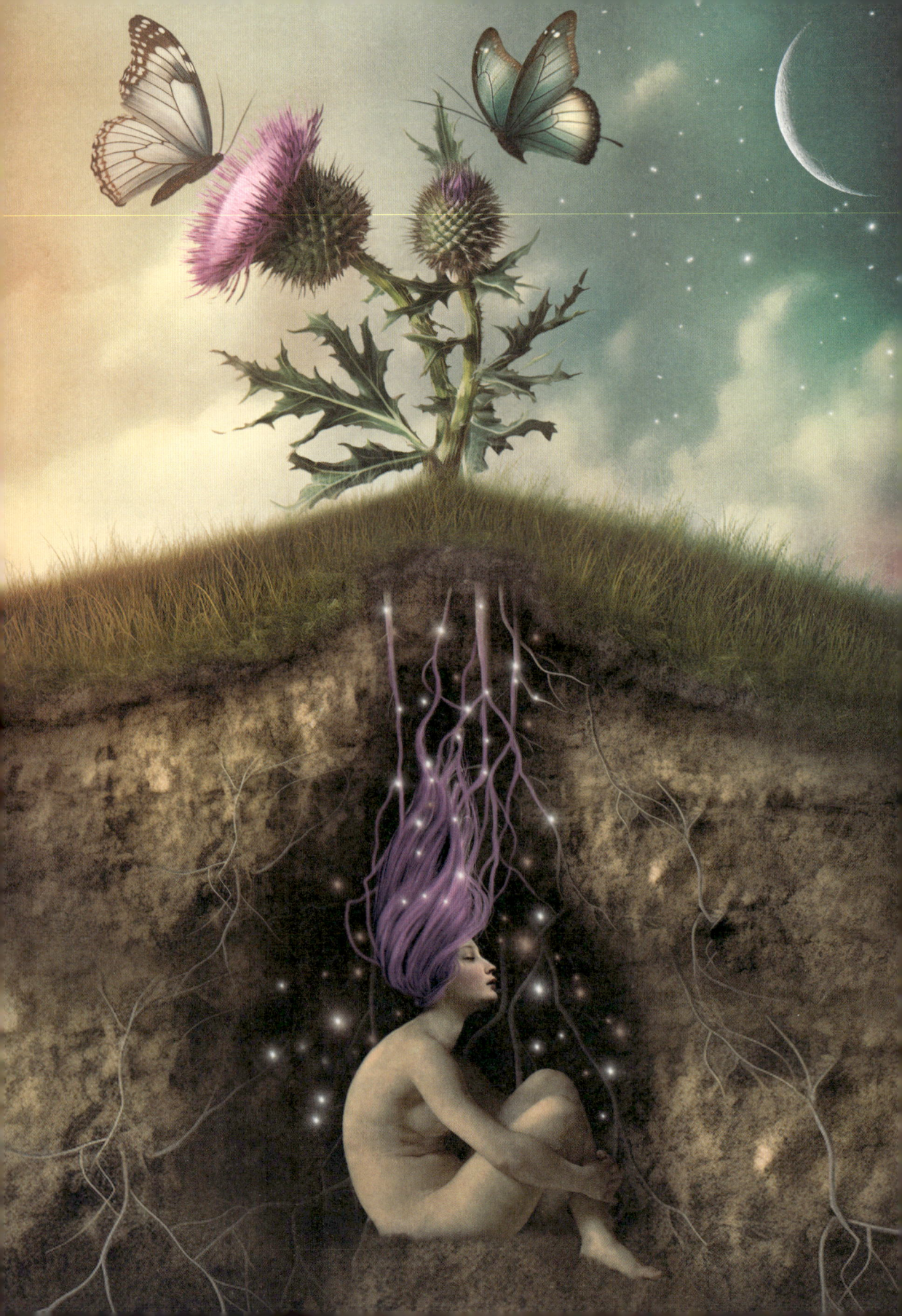

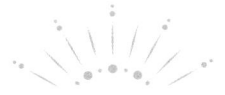

THISTLE

— Cirsium vulgare —

Thistles often grow near houses in the suburbs. They stand out against the sky with stiff, spiny leaves. Before opening, the flower, set atop a tall stem, has thorns, and when it opens it takes on a shape very similar to a small artichoke flower. The leaves and flower receptacles are also a delicacy. When eaten raw, they have a unique flavor that balances sweet and salty, reminiscent of the artichoke. In phytotherapy, you can use thistle for its diuretic and depurating properties, which can support kidney health; the leaves and roots, when used for infusions or herbal teas, help eliminate toxins and promote diuresis. In many traditions, the thistle is considered a symbol of protection. Its thorns are believed to keep away evil spirits and unwanted intruders. It is often used in magical preparations to repel negative energy, create energy barriers, and promote mental clarity.

– MAGICAL USES –

*Due to its **thorny nature**, the thistle is associated with protective abilities and repelling negative energy. The thistle was believed to **protect against snakes**. Keeping a dried thistle flower in one's pocket protects not only from snakes but **also from evildoers**. In addition, it gives strength and vigor.*

Little Magical Protection Ritual

YOU WILL NEED:

- *1 bunch of dried wild thistle or a few fresh leaves*
- *1 ribbon or one strand of white or purple wool*
- *1 small cloth bag*

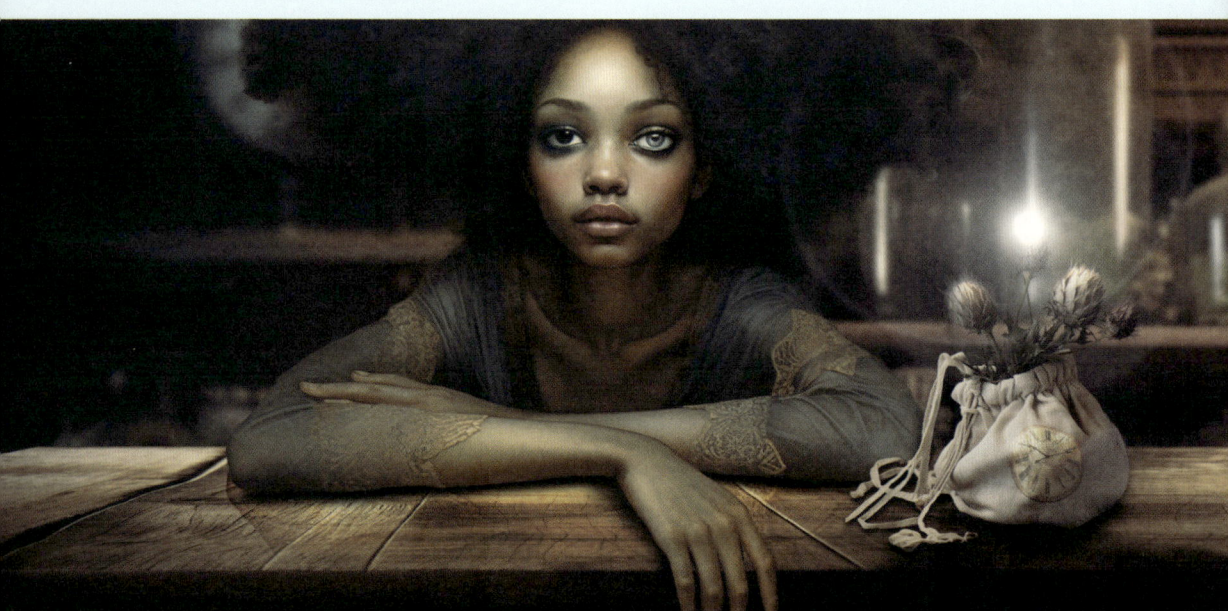

Take the bunch of dried wild thistle or fresh leaves and place them in front of you; focus for a moment on the intention of creating a protective barrier around you. Visualize a halo of white or purple light enveloping you or the area you wish to protect. Take the ribbon or thread of white or purple wool and begin to weave it around the bunch of wild thistle. Meanwhile, say your intention out loud or in your head; you can recite a simple formula, such as *"With the power of the wild thistle, I create a wall of protection around me (or around the specific place). I am safe and protected from all negativity."* After weaving the ribbon or thread around the wild thistle bunch, take the cloth bag and place the bunch inside. Close the bag and tie the ribbon or thread around the end to seal it. You can keep it with you or hang it at the entrance to your home as an amulet of protection. If you wish, you can also take it with you to situations or places where you feel that you need extra security. Remember to thank the thistle energy, perhaps leaving a small gift where you picked it.

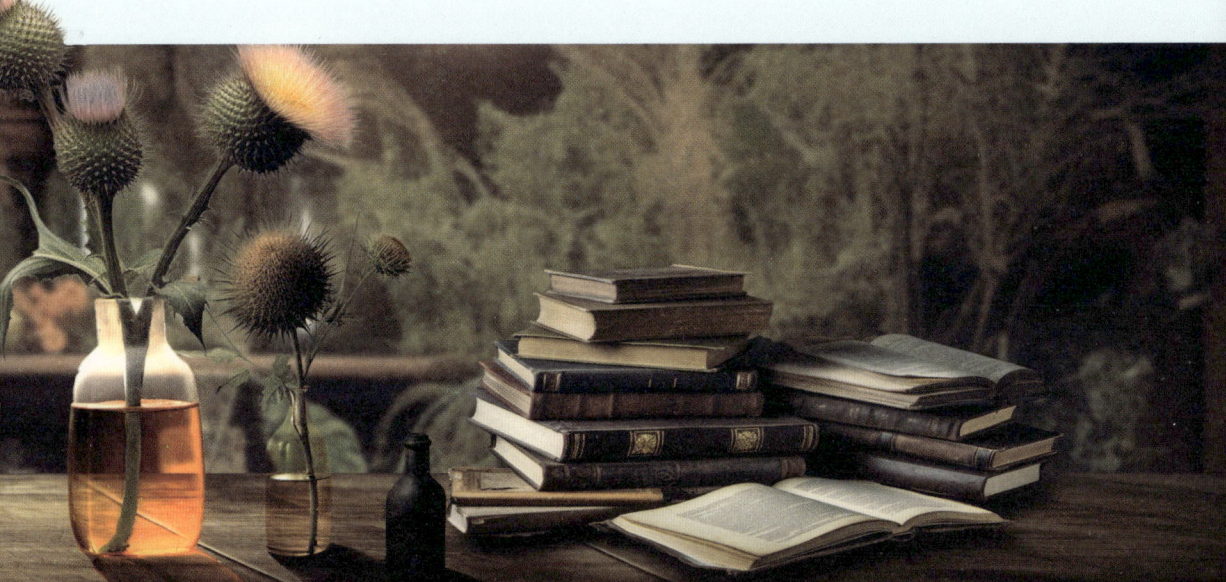

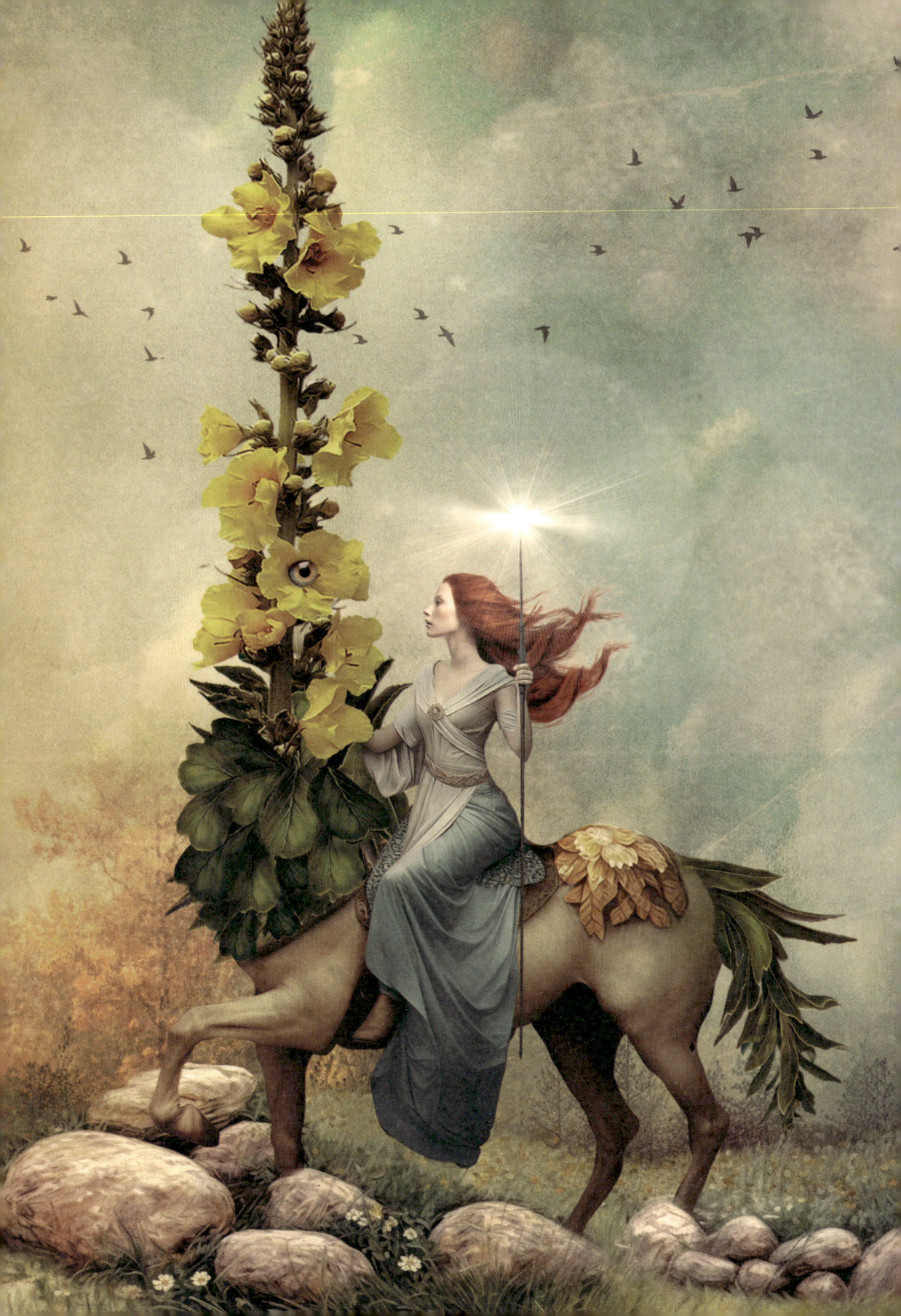

GREAT MULLEIN

– Verbascum thapsus –

In the middle of summer, great mullein explodes into a flurry of yellow flowers, arranged on the plant as if they were a flame. Not surprisingly, this plant was also used as light, soaked in oil and lit. It is nicknamed candlewick due to the fluff of its leaves, which were turned into wicks and used in candles. Its velvety leaves, when dried and infused, produce a soothing tea renowned for its respiratory benefits; however, it is important to filter the herbal tea very well to remove the fluff, which is an irritant. The oily macerate obtained from mullein flowers offers a potent remedy for ear infections that relieves pain. From a magical point of view, the plant is linked to courage, sunshine, and the ability to overcome darkness; it can be worn or carried to promote love and can be placed in a pouch and under a pillow to repel nightmares.

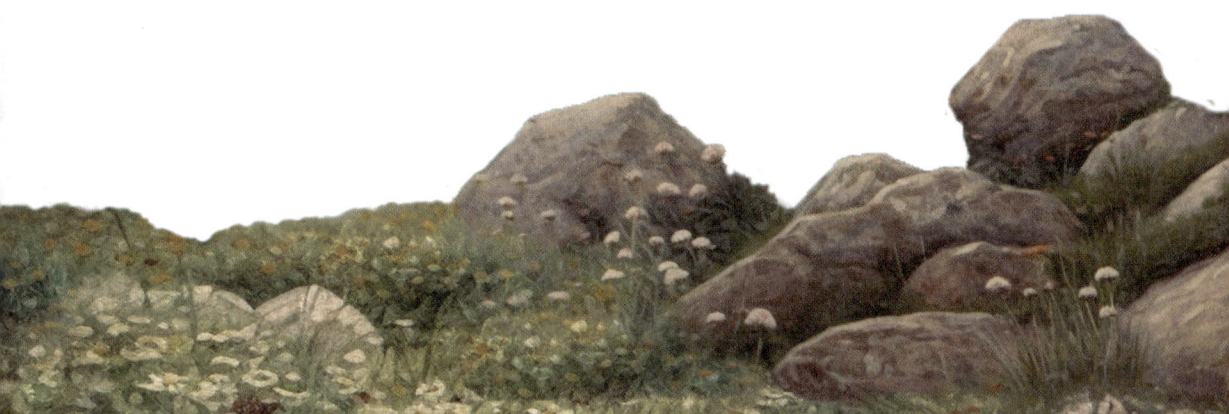

– COSMETIC USES –

*One of the most popular ways to use great mullein in cosmetics is as a facial toner. Its infusion acts as a **gentle astringent**, helping to tighten pores, balance skin pH, and promote a radiant complexion. To create a mullein tonic, place a handful of mullein flowers in boiling water and let it steep for about ten minutes. Let the infusion cool, strain it, and store it in a clean bottle. Apply the tonic to your face with a cotton ball, gently wiping it over your skin for a truly radiant result. Mullein can also be used on hair. Steeping mullein flowers in a carrier oil like coconut or jojoba oil creates a nourishing elixir that **contributes to hair and scalp care**. Fill a glass jar with dried mullein flowers and cover them with your chosen carrier oil, then seal the jar tightly and let it sit in a cool, dark place for two to three weeks. Strain the oil to remove the flowers, and store it in a dark glass jar. To use, massage a few drops of this oil onto the scalp and distribute it over the hair, leaving it to deeply moisturize and revitalize the hair.*

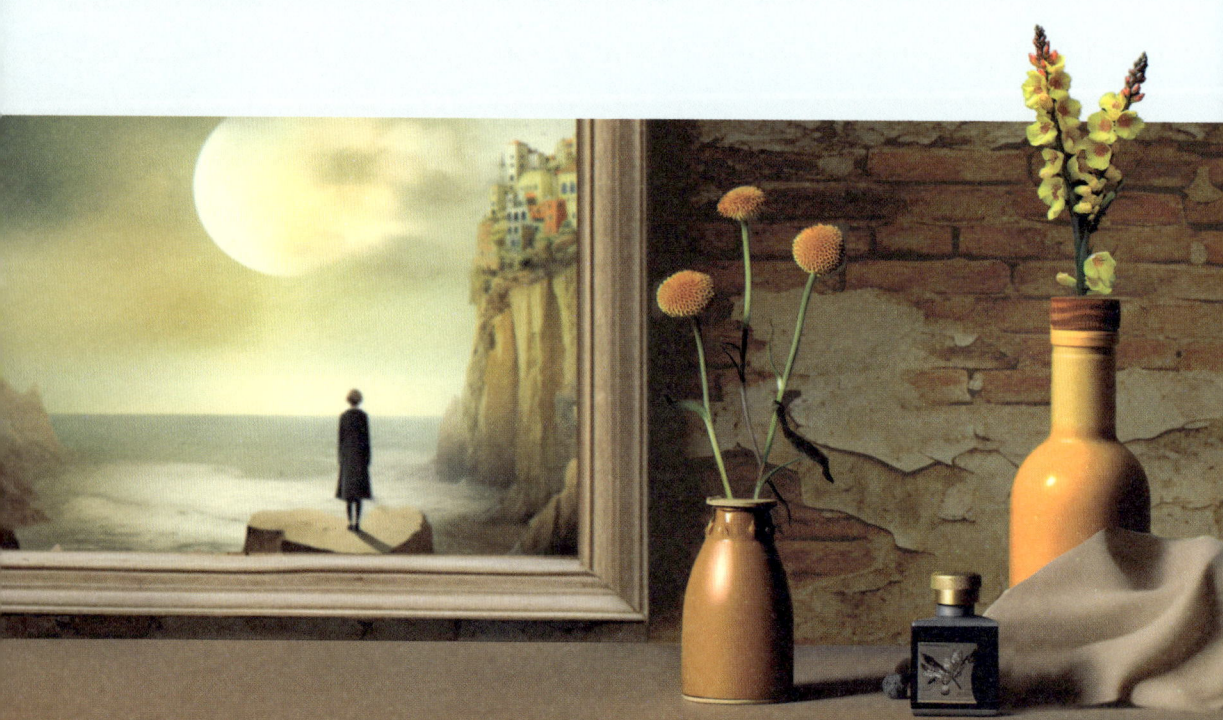

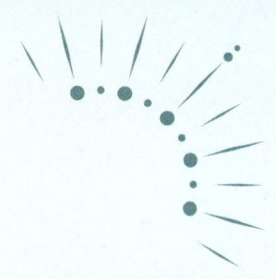

Mullein
Lip Balm

YOU WILL NEED:

- *1 spoonful of shea butter*
- *1 spoonful of coconut oil*
- *1 spoonful of beeswax*
- *1 spoonful of almond oil*
- *1 spoonful of mullein flower oil (previously infused)*

Melt the wax, coconut oil, almond oil, and shea butter in a small saucepan over a double boiler. Once melted, wait for them to cool slightly and then add the mullein oil. Pour it all into a small jar and wait for it to solidify. Now the lip balm is ready! The presence of the oils and the infusion of mullein flowers help protect lips from external agents, keeping them soft and moisturized.

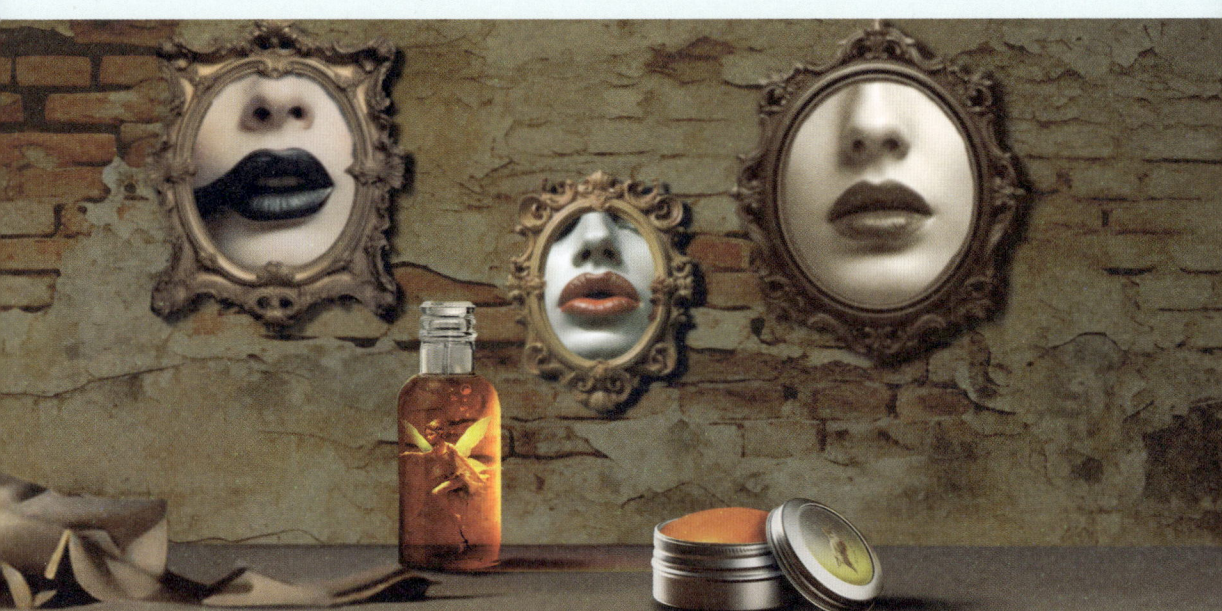

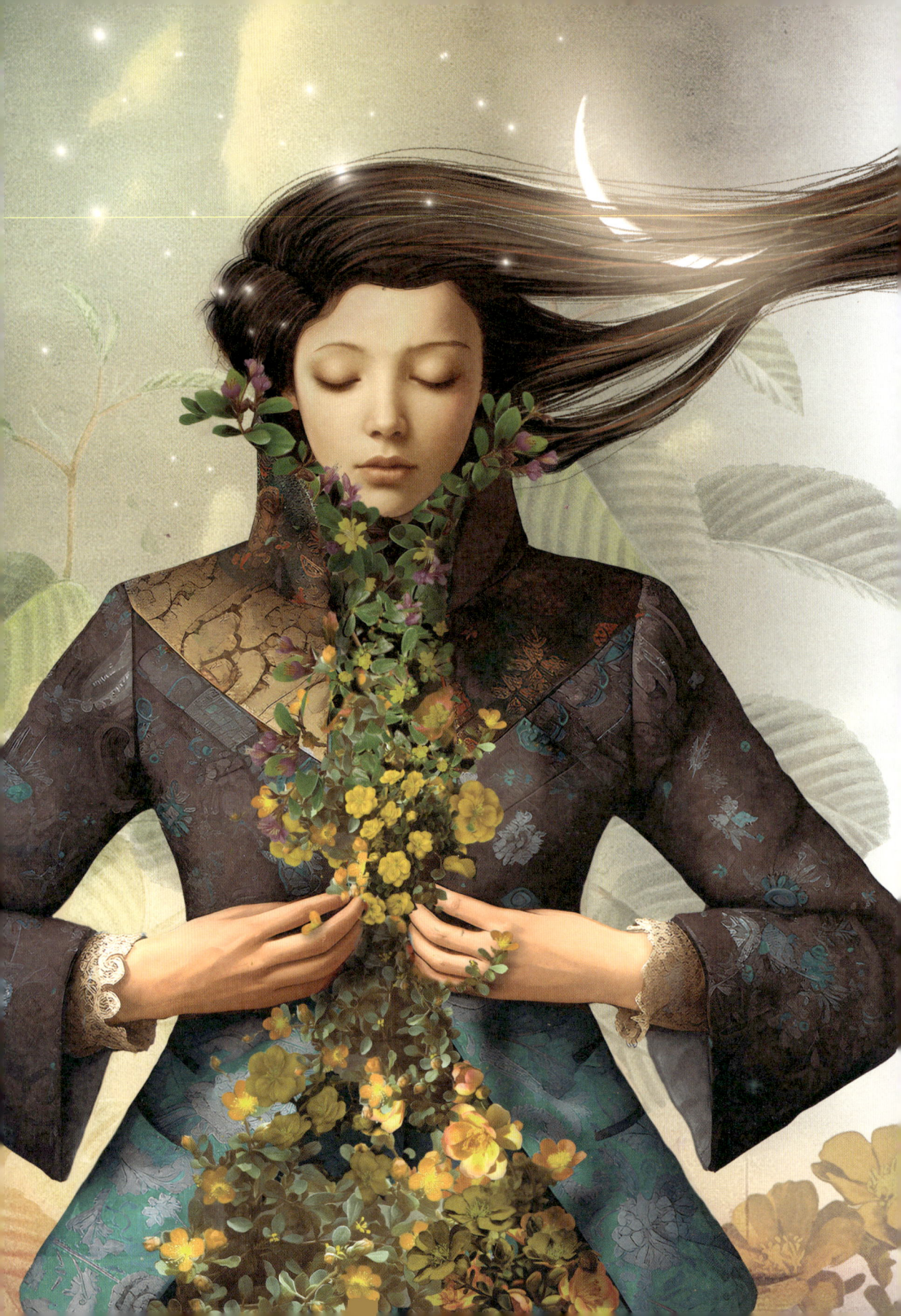

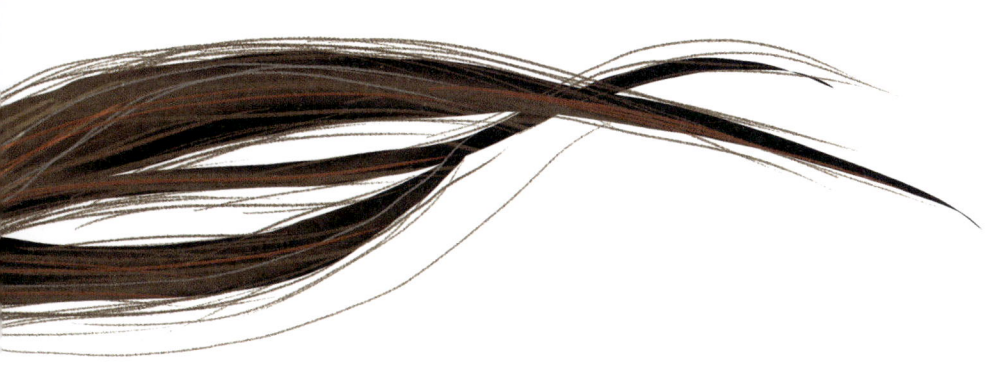

PURSLANE

— Portulaca oleracea —

Purslane is a succulent plant with fleshy, oval, and shiny leaves and reddish stems that grows anywhere, especially if the soil gets a lot of sun and is well drained. Purslane flowers have petals of various shades ranging from white, pink, yellow, and even orange to deep red. There are different types of purslane. Wild purslane often has small, yellow flowers. Its leaves contain good amounts of vitamins A, C, and E, and minerals such as magnesium and potassium, nutrients that help boost the immune system, improve skin and eye health, and promote the body's overall well-being. Its leaves also contain omega-3 fatty acids, which help to control metabolism and have a beneficial effect on cholesterol. It can be eaten raw, has a vaguely tart flavor reminiscent of lemon, and is therefore excellent in salads or alongside raw or cooked vegetables.

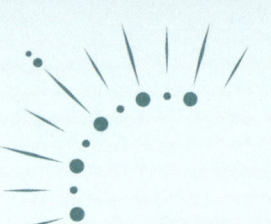

– CULINARY USES –

*The young, tender leaves of purslane can be **added to salads** to give it a fresh touch and a slightly tart flavor. You can simply wash the leaves, gently dry them, and mix them with other crisp greens such as lettuce or cucumbers. Or you can **make a pesto** with the fresh leaves, chopping them with walnuts and garlic and adding extra virgin olive oil. A tasty way to preserve and use this plant is to **pickle the leaves**.*

Pickled Purslane

YOU WILL NEED:

- *Fresh and clean purslane leaves*
- *Apple cider vinegar or white wine vinegar**
- *Salt*
- *Garlic*
- *Spices to taste (like mustard seeds, coriander seeds, or chili pepper)*

Sterilize a glass jar and lid by boiling them in water for a few minutes. Let them cool, then fill the sterilized jar with well-washed purslane leaves, leaving some free space at the top. Finally, add chopped garlic and spices to taste. In a pot, bring the vinegar to a boil along with the salt. Once it reaches the boiling point, turn off the heat and let it cool for a few minutes. Gently pour the hot vinegar into the jar, completely covering the purslane leaves. Seal the jar tightly with the lid and let it cool. Keep the jar in the refrigerator for at least a week before consuming the purslane pickles so that all the flavors will blend to perfection. You can use it in sandwiches and salads, or on vegetables. Remember that once the jar is opened, the pickles should be eaten in a week.

*You should completely cover the purslane leaves in the jar with vinegar. The amount of vinegar will then depend on the size of the jar and the amount of leaves you have on hand. The amount of salt will be about two teaspoons per cup of vinegar.

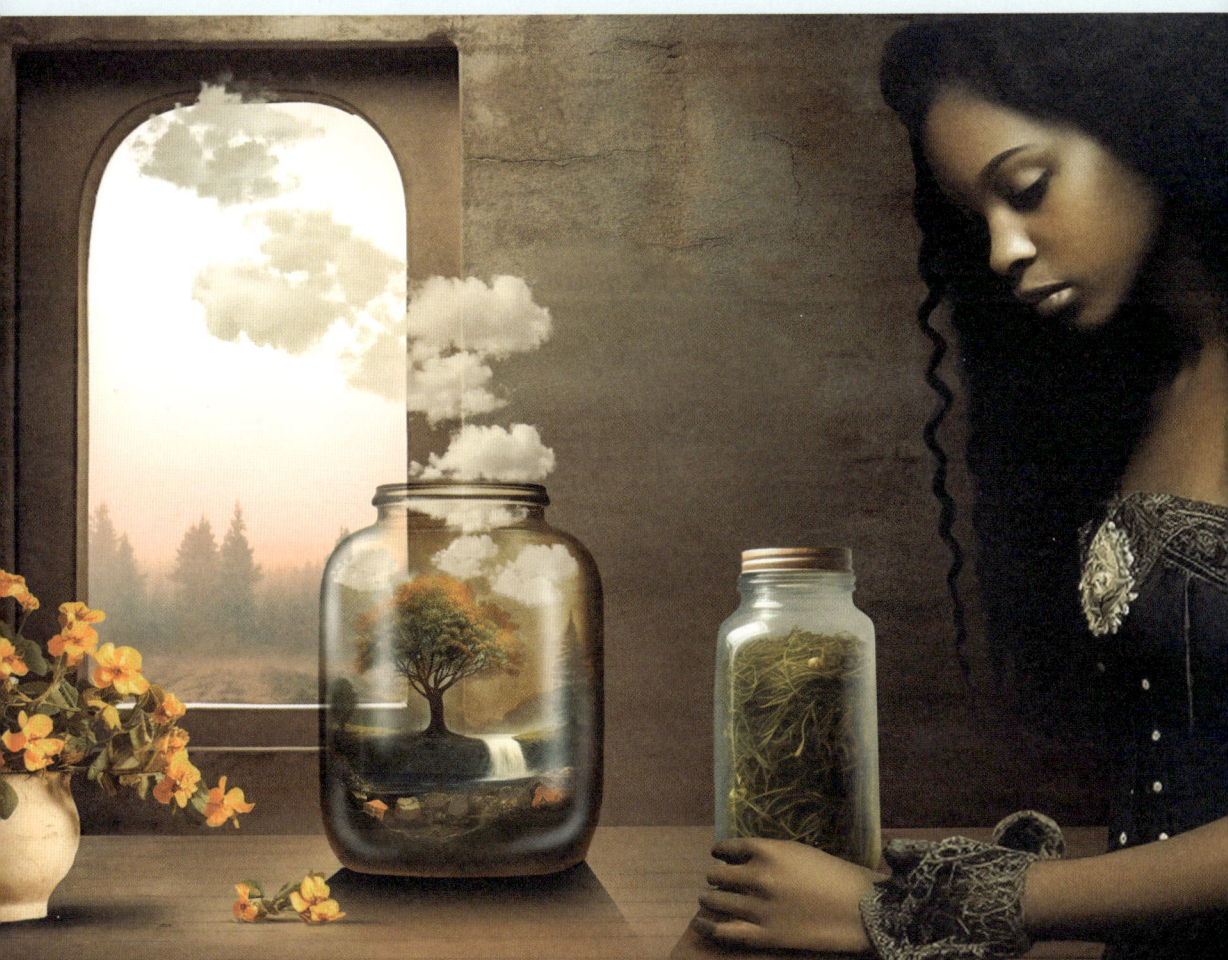

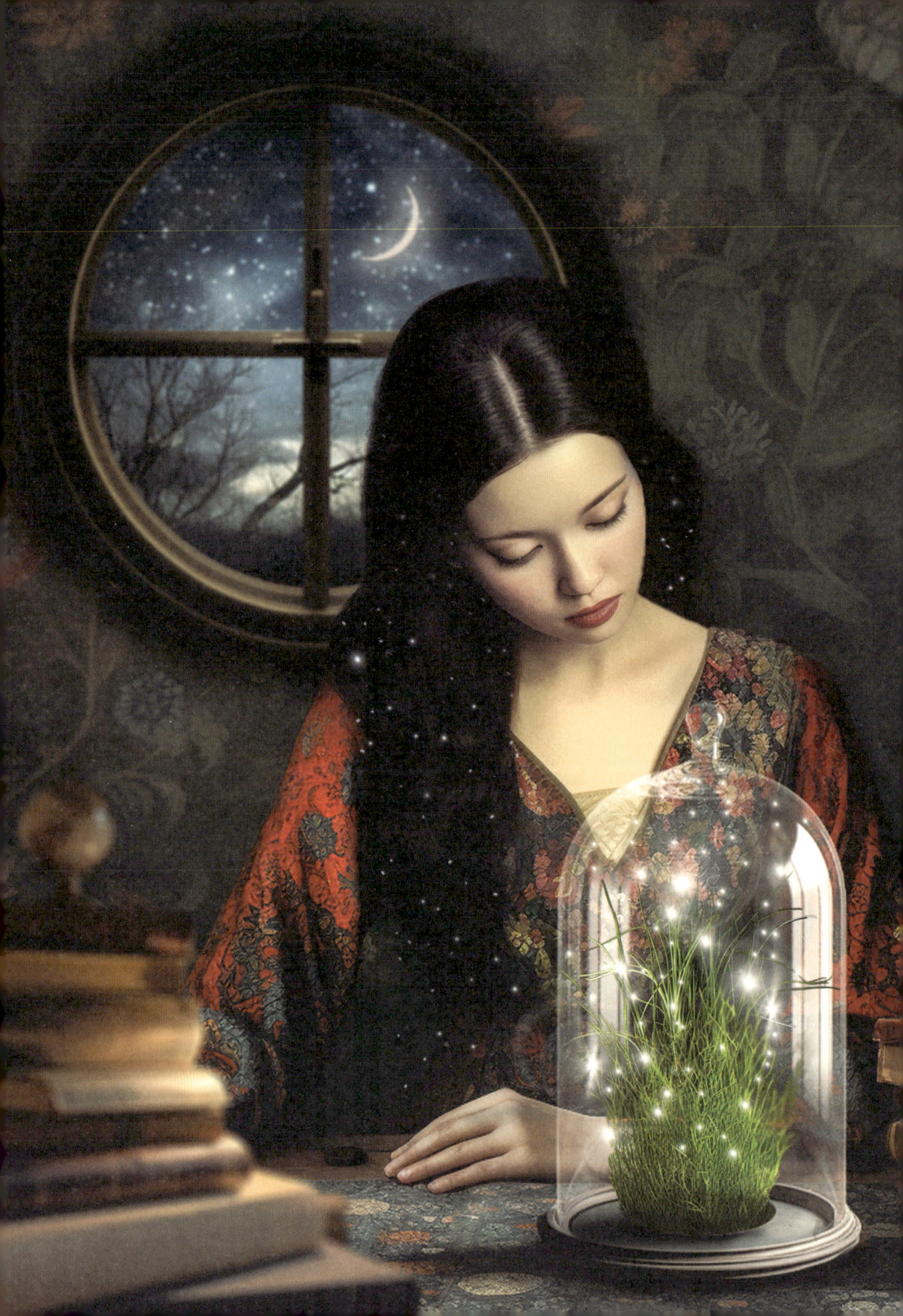

WITCHGRASS

— AGROPYRON REPENS —

Witchgrass is the quintessential weed. Often hated, it is plucked from yards and vegetable gardens because of its weedy and invasive nature. Yet Nobel Prize–winning poet Louise Glück dedicated a wonderful poem to it entitled "Witchgrass," in which the plant becomes a symbol of persistence and resilience, an emblem of the life force inherent in nature. The poem is a eulogy to the vitality and resilience of witchgrass, which is also rich in phytotherapeutic properties. Its roots are used to prepare herbal teas and infusions with diuretic and anti-inflammatory properties. Witchgrass can play an important role in soil stabilization due to its fibrous roots that help prevent erosion. In addition, its ability to withstand harsh environmental conditions makes it a hardy plant that can contribute to biodiversity in degraded habitats.

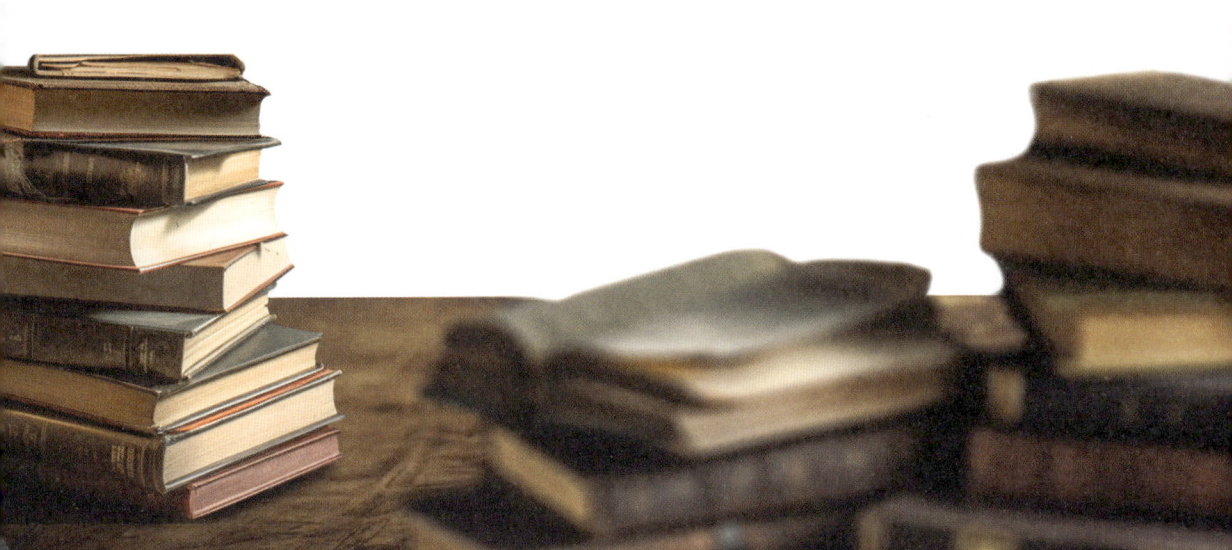

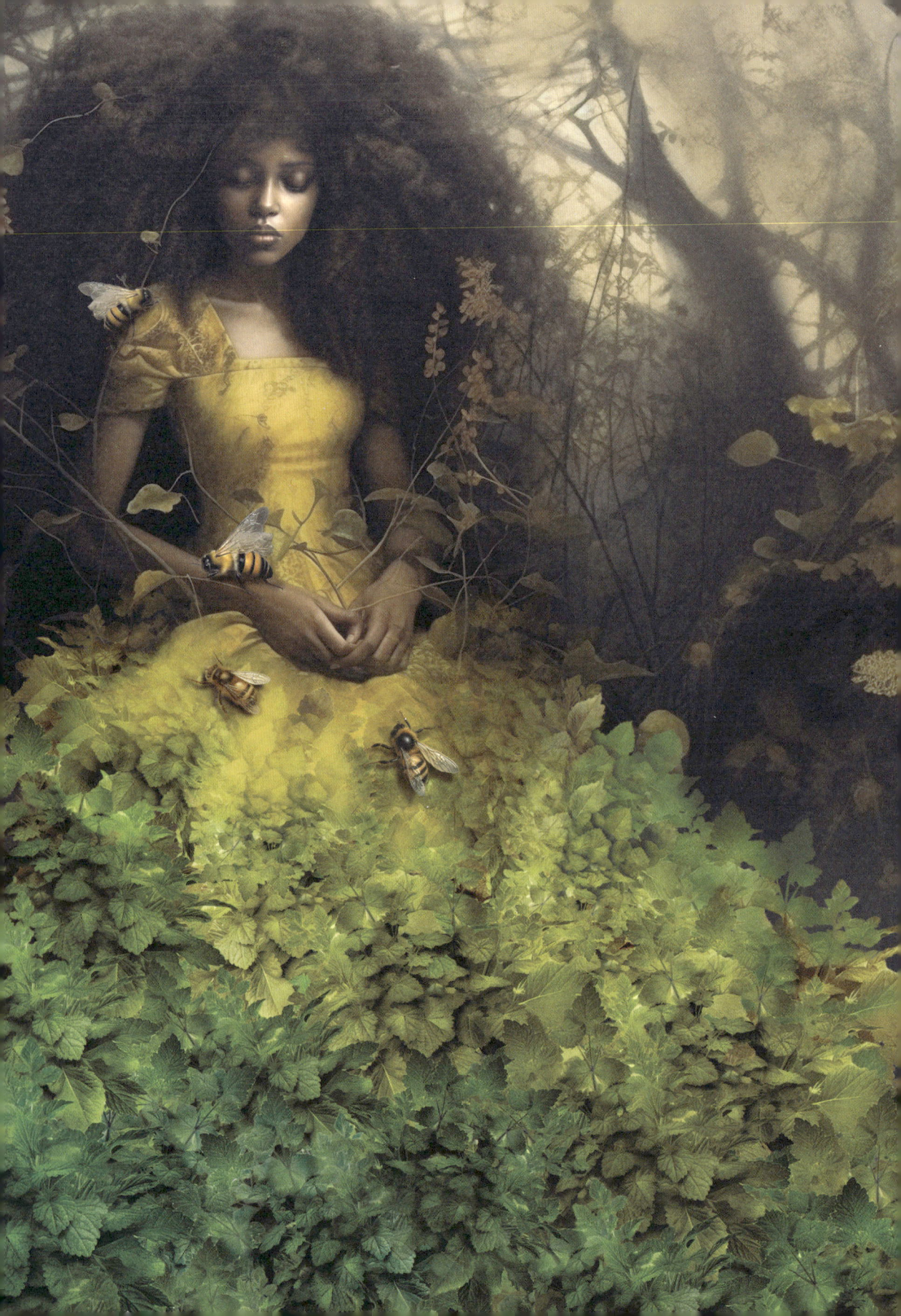

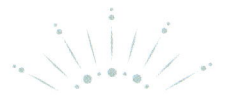

LEMON BALM

— MELISSA OFFICINALIS —

The history of lemon balm is closely linked to the world of bees. Bees seem to be attracted to the plant's aromas; therefore, it has been customary since ancient times to rub the plant's leaves on the hives so that the swarms remain captivated by its aroma and do not escape. The name of the plant, *Melissa,* is derived from the Greek word for bee. The word also has symbolic meaning: in Greek mythology, *Melissa* was the name of the nymph who raised a young Jupiter on honey. We can therefore already glimpse the qualities of sweetness and gentleness inherent in this plant, which is used in herbal tea both as a central nervous system soother and to promote good sleep. In addition, lemon balm has excellent antispasmodic and digestive abilities, and can foster a good mood, modulating emotions related to well-being in general. On a more subtle level, it is connected to a sense of welcoming, feeling at home, and childhood.

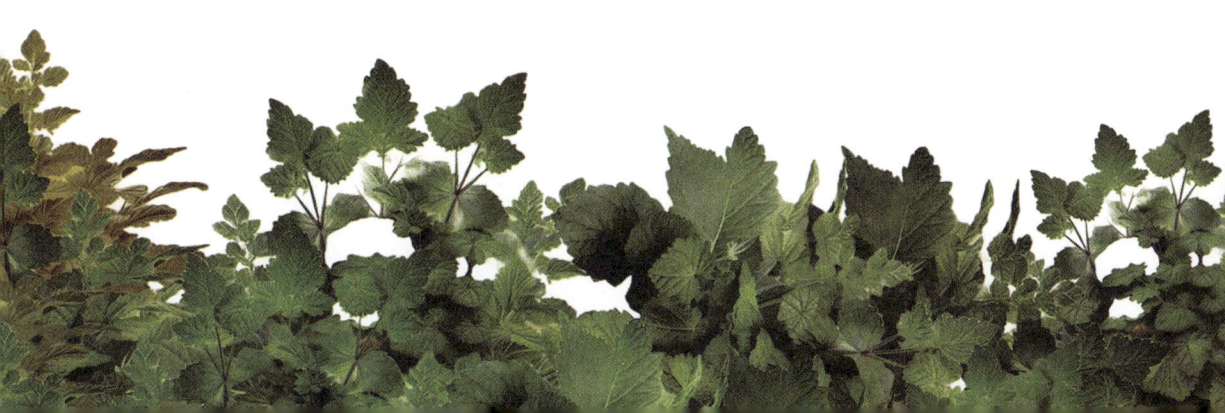

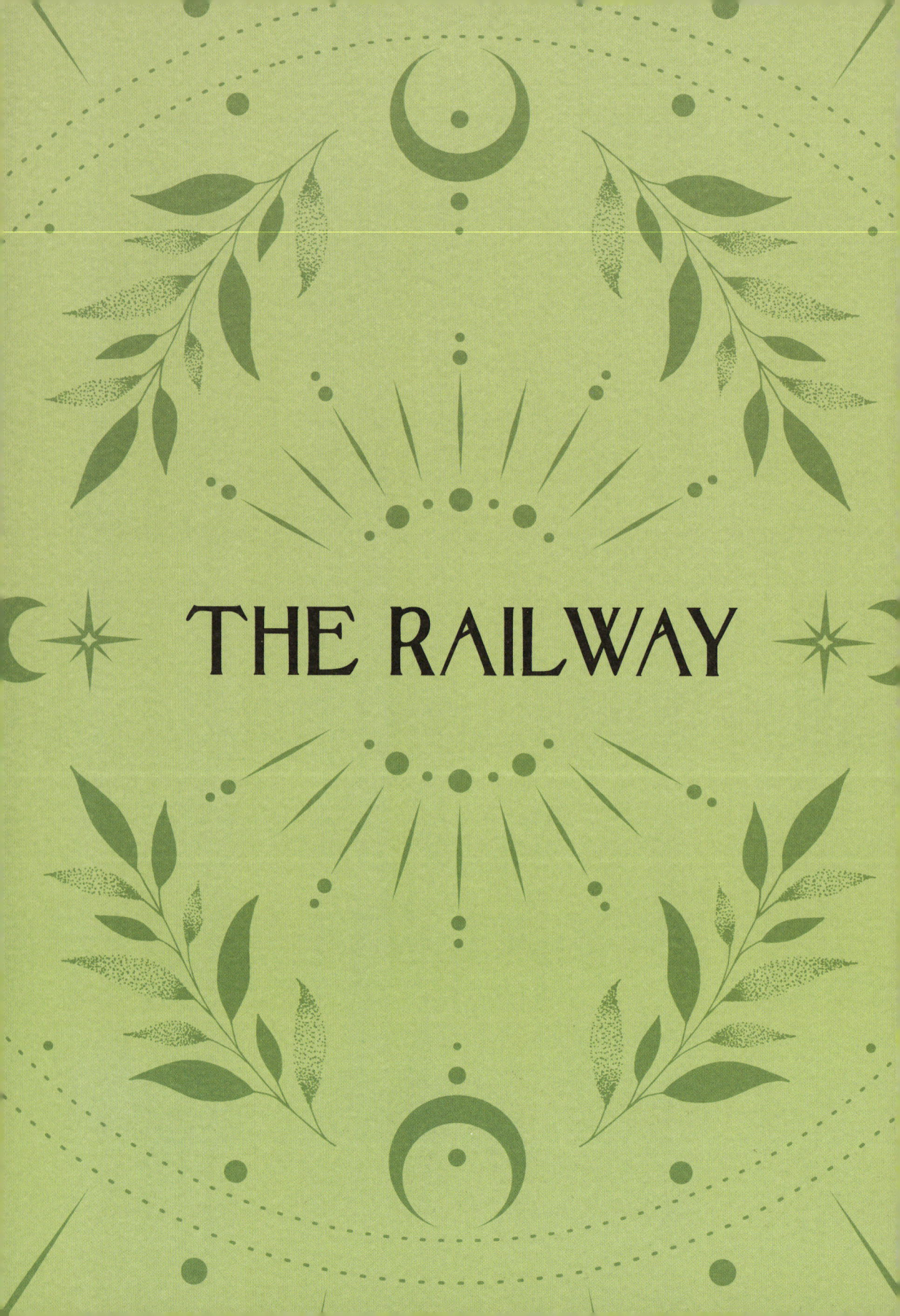

THE RAILWAY

The abandoned railway winds through the countryside and down a trail that seems to wander off into the horizon. The rusted tracks are now a refuge for wild grasses and shrubs, climbing along the edges as if to hold together what remains of a lost world. If you take the path along the tracks, you will encounter a few peeling ivy-covered walls. You can read the old signs marking deserted stations, in the shade of which blue mallow and chickweed grow. There is an air of magic here. The secrets of children lie there, like little colored pebbles hidden under the steps and wild caper plants, growing undisturbed inside the cracks in the walls. Saint-John's-wort grows lushly along the edges of the tracks, while chamomile climbs the red brick walls of the old stations. Rusty tracks are fantastic roads to other worlds, a map for the imagination. Along the track, witches gather in search of wild herbs to use in their magical rituals. The railway is a place of meeting and exchange. The seeds of weeds arrive there, carried by the wind, witches by magic. Here, mingling with ordinary people, witches gather poppy seeds or trace runes in the air to protect the journey. The railroad is like a portal to a new world, traveling down the paths marked by tracks and dreams; it is here that crossroads meet, places sacred to witches as places of power. As Fannie Flagg wrote in her book *Fried Green Tomatoes at the Whistle Stop Cafe*, the railroad has the power to transport the dreams, illusions, hopes, and disappointments of all humanity down its tracks. And it is this power, perhaps, that makes it such a magical and fascinating place.

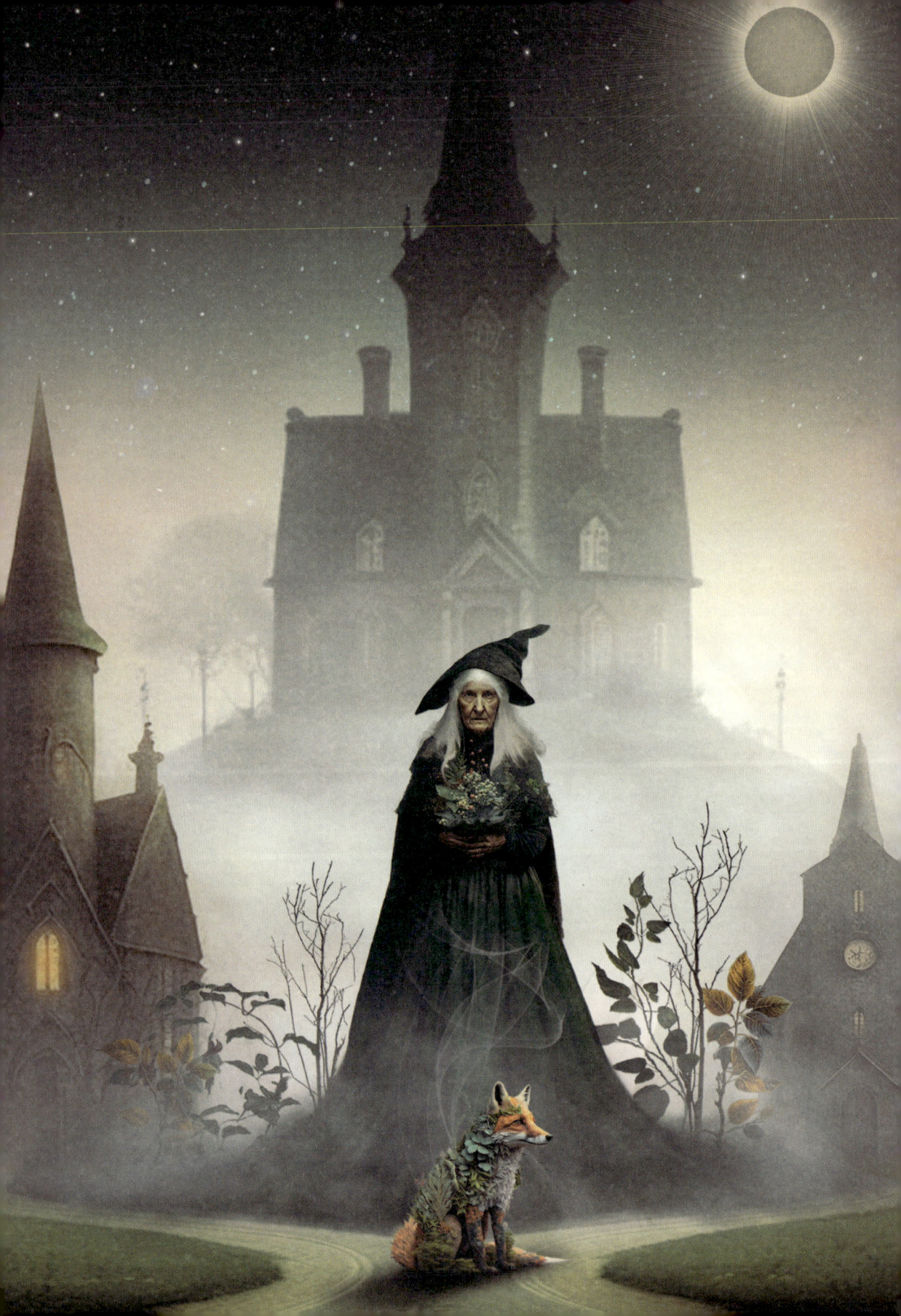

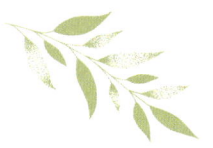
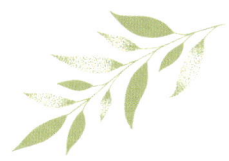

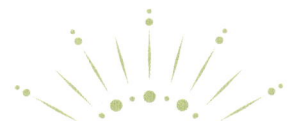

THE WITCH
OF THE CROSSROADS

—

The crossroads is an intersection
of four roads. It is always a magical
place, linked to the choice and power
of taking the right path. At the center,
you often find natural altars or shrines
of sacred figures. The crossroads,
the subject of numerous legends and
superstitions, is considered the place
where the material world and the
spiritual world meet in many cultures.

It is associated with several deities and mythological figures, including Hecate, the Greek goddess of magic and night, often depicted with three heads representing the three phases of the moon and the three realms of life (earth, sky, and sea). Hecate, who also embodies the three ages of the goddess (maiden, adult, and elder), is a triple goddess. Because of this nature, she is probably connected to the intersection of multiple paths.

In some folk traditions, the crossroads is believed to be a meeting place for witches, who hold their nightly *sabbaths* there and offer sacrifices to spirits. According to some beliefs, walking with your head hanging down over a crossroads can bring good luck, while getting stuck in the middle attracts bad luck.

In some esoteric traditions, the crossroads is seen as a transition point between life and death, between the old and the new, and represents a choice between different directions and paths in life. It is here that the crossroads witch dwells. A mythical character often found in fairy tales and fantasy stories, she is the one who asks riddles to be solved and meddles, for better or worse, in the hero's journey. According to tradition, the crossroads witch has the power to control nature spirits and manipulate the forces of life and death.

She is often described as a lonely, elderly woman who wears disheveled clothing and a pointed hat.

Daughter of Hecate, priestess of the moon, her knowledge of medicinal plants and the secrets of magic make her a respected figure to be sought after for her herbal wisdom. Her being is reminiscent of the Celtic traditions of Avalon and its priestesses, who lived on the Isle of Apples to learn the magical arts. But she also harkens back to the fairy-tale tradition of the old woman who lives at the edge of the woods, the old woman of herbs, the witch who heals and who, through an initiation, allows the hero to grow and continue on the path.

> The crossroads witch is an expert gatherer, and her magic feeds on those traveling herbs found along abandoned tracks. They are herbs that maintain a link to the dimension of travel and expansion, and the resulting magical preparations are thus about protection and discovery.

A priestess of nature, this witch is an expert in spells of protection for travelers who pass by her station, who can see her silhouetted in the distance along the rusted tracks. A fox sits by her side, and she holds a bunch of mugwort and hawthorn. The scent of wild herbs reaches you, traveler. Put a mugwort leaf in a shoe, listen to what it whispers to you, and it will protect you along the journey.

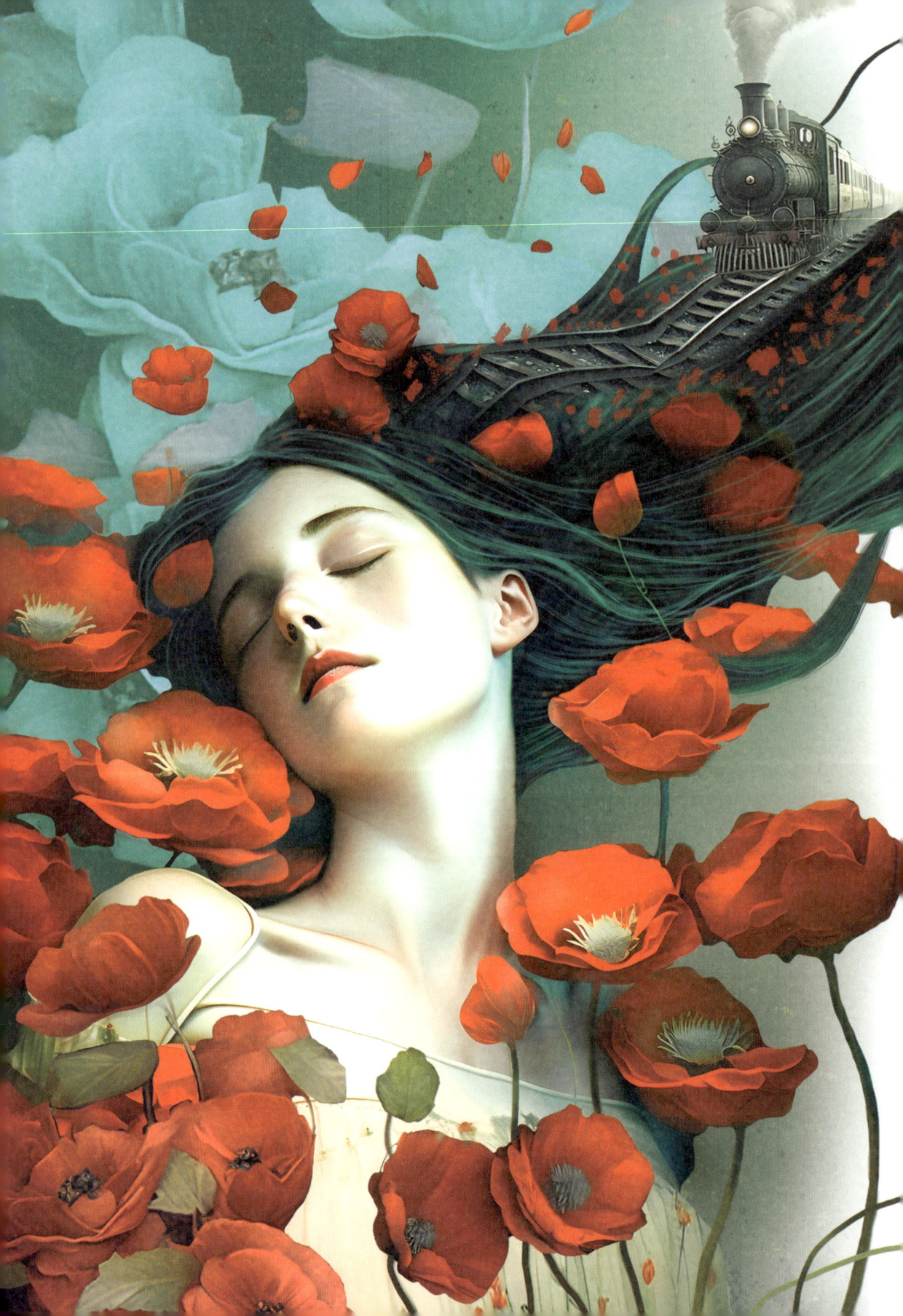

WILD POPPY

— Papaver rhoeas —

Along railroad tracks in spring, it is very easy to see red poppies dancing in the wind. Their deep red has inspired poets and painters, and it is a wonder to watch them bloom. Poppy is none other than the wild poppy (*Papaver rhoeas*), different from the opium poppy (*Papaver somniferum*), which is much taller and has purple petals, and its latex is a potent mixture of the powerful alkaloid opium. Wild poppy is known for its calming and sedative properties and is often used as a natural remedy to soothe coughs. The dried petals can be used in herbal teas. Wild poppy extract is also used as an ingredient in many skin-care products because of its soothing and anti-inflammatory properties. From a magical point of view, wild poppy has protective properties related to love and dreams. Putting a handful of its petals inside your pillow will spark prophetic dreams.

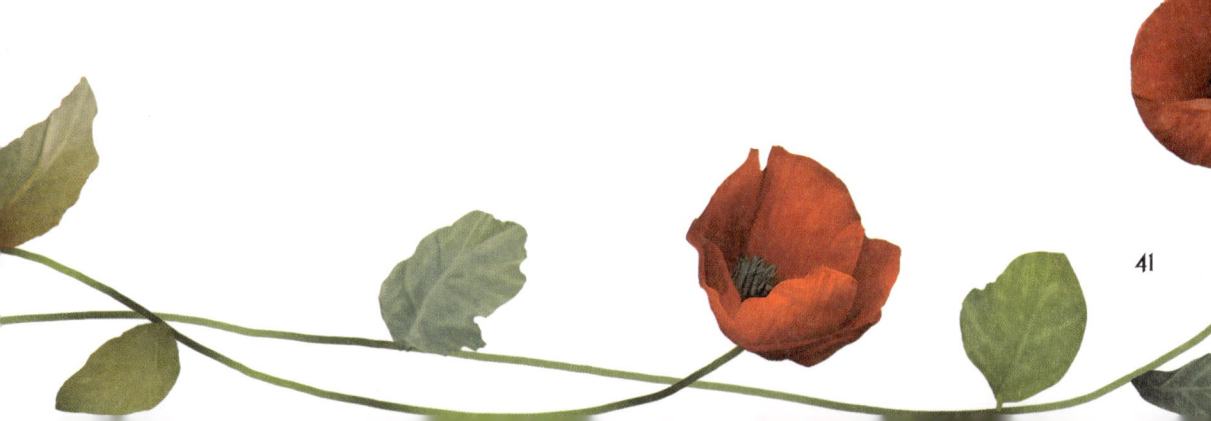

Nourishing Wild Poppy Hand and Face Cream

*This nourishing wild poppy hand and face cream is **ideal for dry and dehydrated skin**, thanks to the emollient and nourishing properties of poppy petals and shea butter.*

YOU WILL NEED:

- 1 spoonful of dried wild poppy petals
- 2 spoonfuls of shea butter
- 1 spoonful of sunflower seed oil
- 5 drops of lavender essential oil

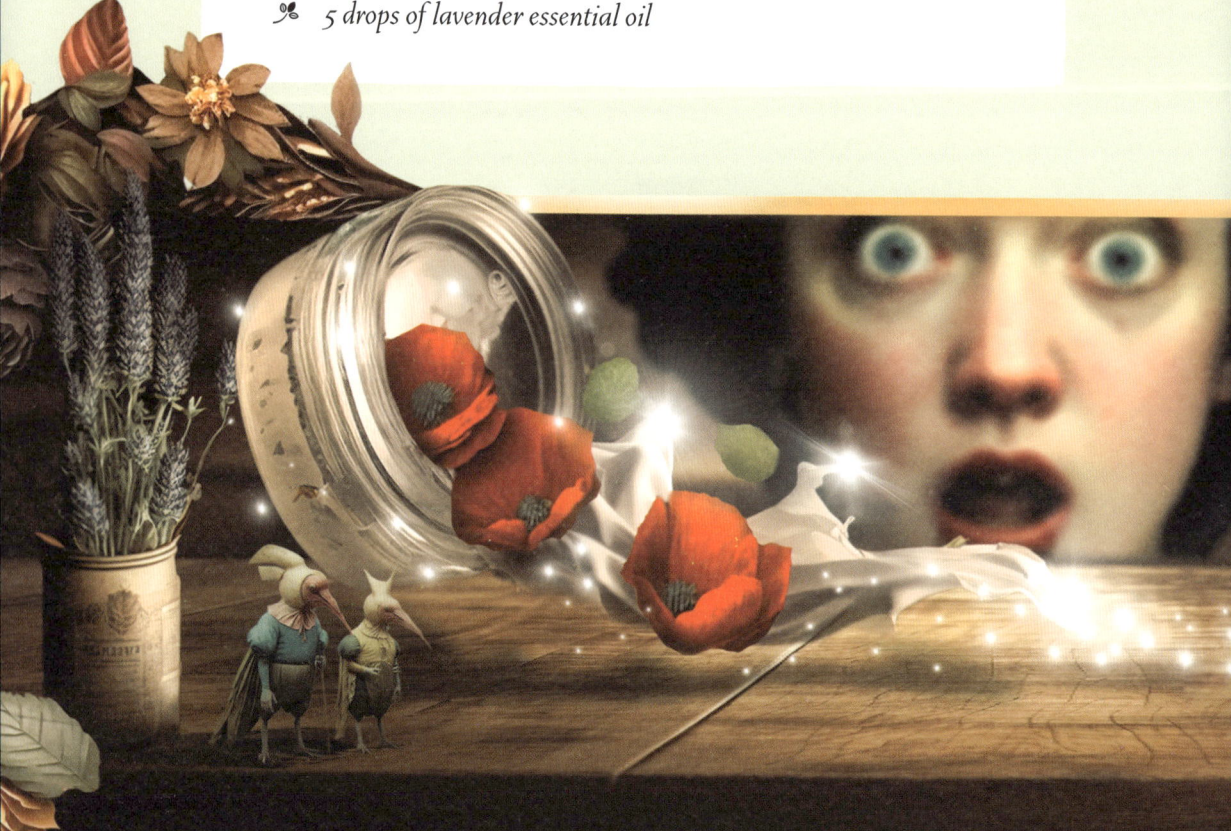

Grind the dried wild poppy petals into a fine powder using a coffee grinder or mortar. Melt the shea butter in a double boiler. Pour the sunflower seed oil into the bowl containing the shea butter, and mix well. Then add the wild poppy petal powder to the butter-oil mixture and mix again. Finally, add the lavender essential oil and mix well. Pour the resulting cream into a dark glass jar and store in the refrigerator. Use it within two to three weeks.

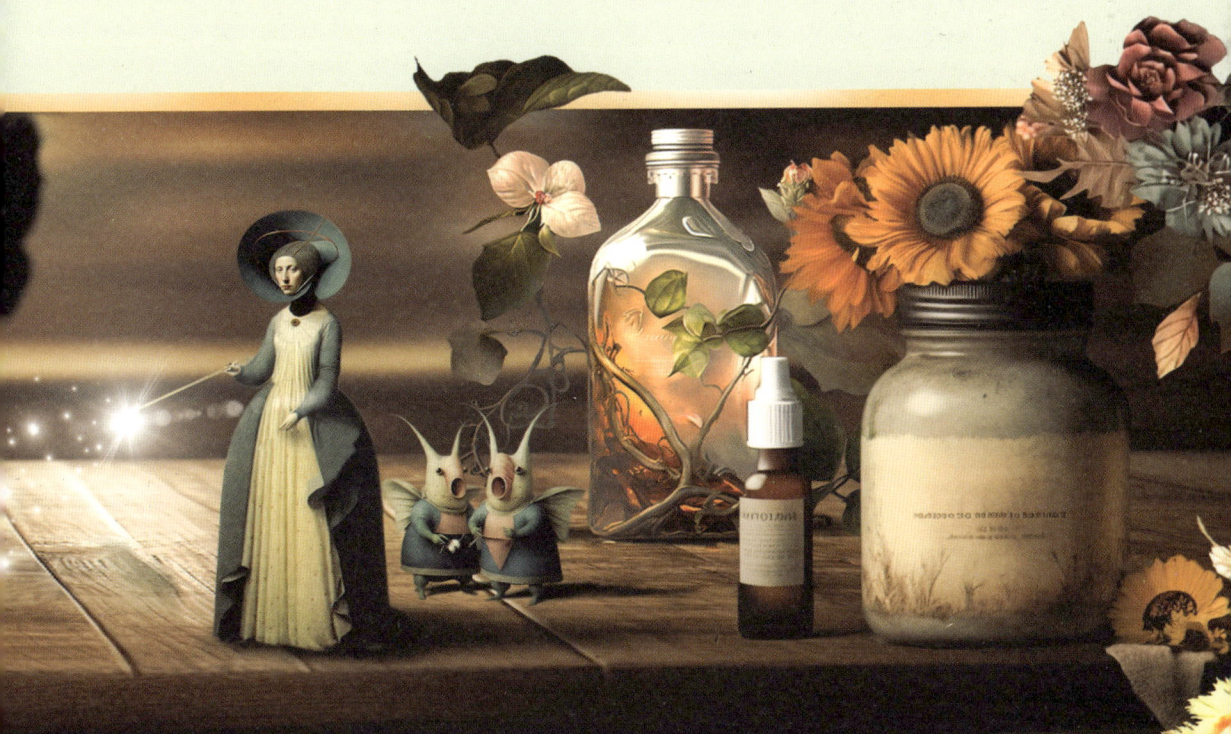

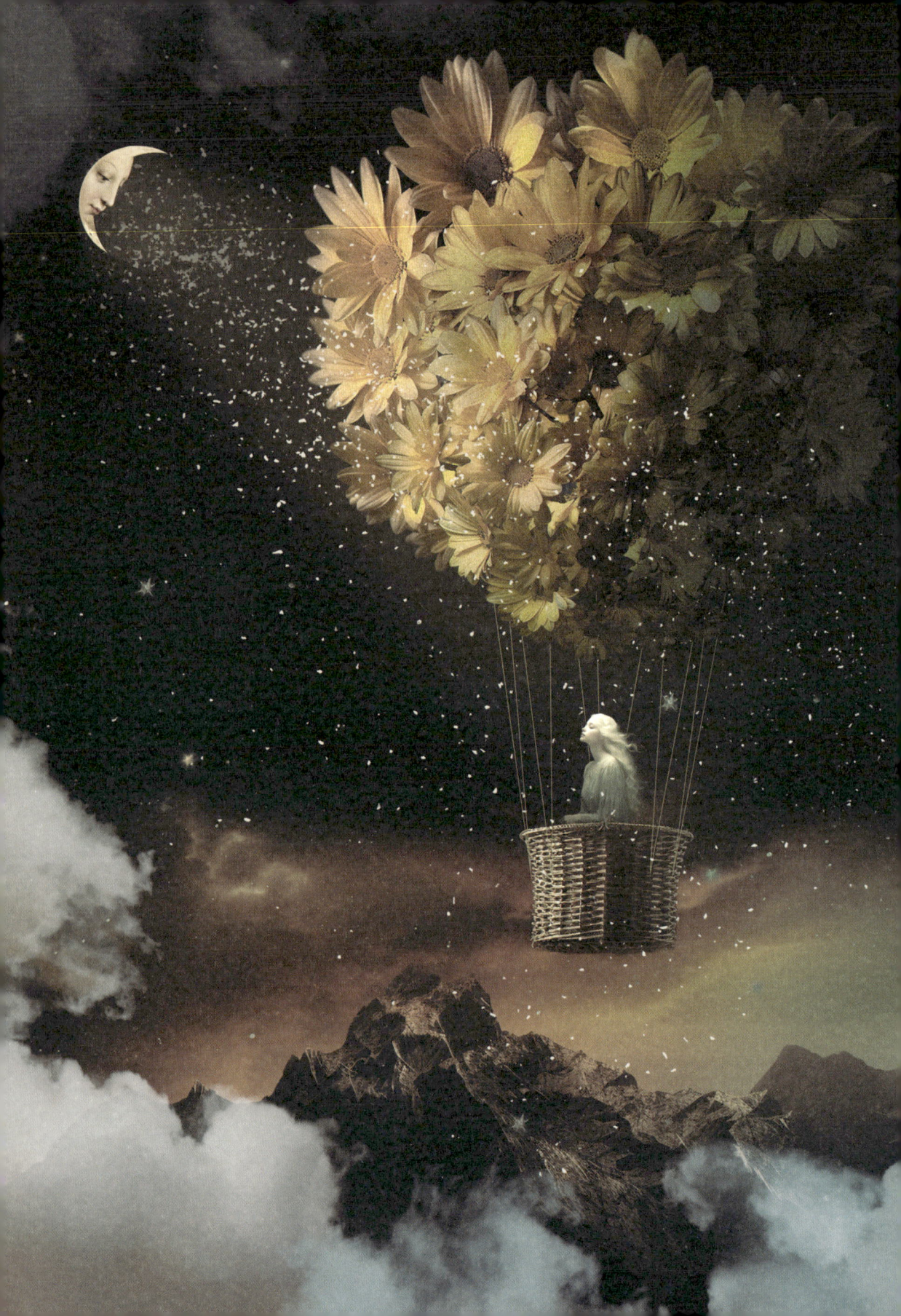

SUNCHOKE

— Helianthus tuberosus —

Sunchoke is a sunny plant that holds its most precious treasure under the ground. Botanically, it is also known as *Helianthus tuberosus* and belongs to the Compositae family. The plant grows and branches with great majesty, reaching considerable heights with its sturdy, gnarled stems. The deep-green leaves stand out against the sky, and the yellow flower brings cheer. The part that is harvested, however, is the tuberous rhizome, which is extracted in the fall, when the plant has faded. Since ancient times, it has been used for its beneficial properties. The roots are rich in inulin, a valuable carbohydrate that supports digestive health and promotes the growth of balanced intestinal flora. In addition, it is edible and tastes great, a mix between a potato and an artichoke. Sunchoke calls to being rooted, to our ability to feel at home and to draw nourishment from what makes us happy.

– CULINARY USES –

*The most delicious part of the sunchoke, also known as the Jerusalem artichoke, is in its roots. Once harvested and cleaned, they reveal a sweet flavor and a slightly crunchy texture, **similar to a carrot or potato**. Nutritionally, sunchokes are a real powerhouse of benefits. Thanks to its inulin content, sunchoke can be useful for diabetics, as it can reduce blood sugar levels. In addition, it **contains vitamins, minerals, and antioxidants** that help strengthen the immune system and promote overall health. You can use it for risottos or cook it with roasted potatoes. It becomes a **great side dish** and makes any combination truly delicious.*

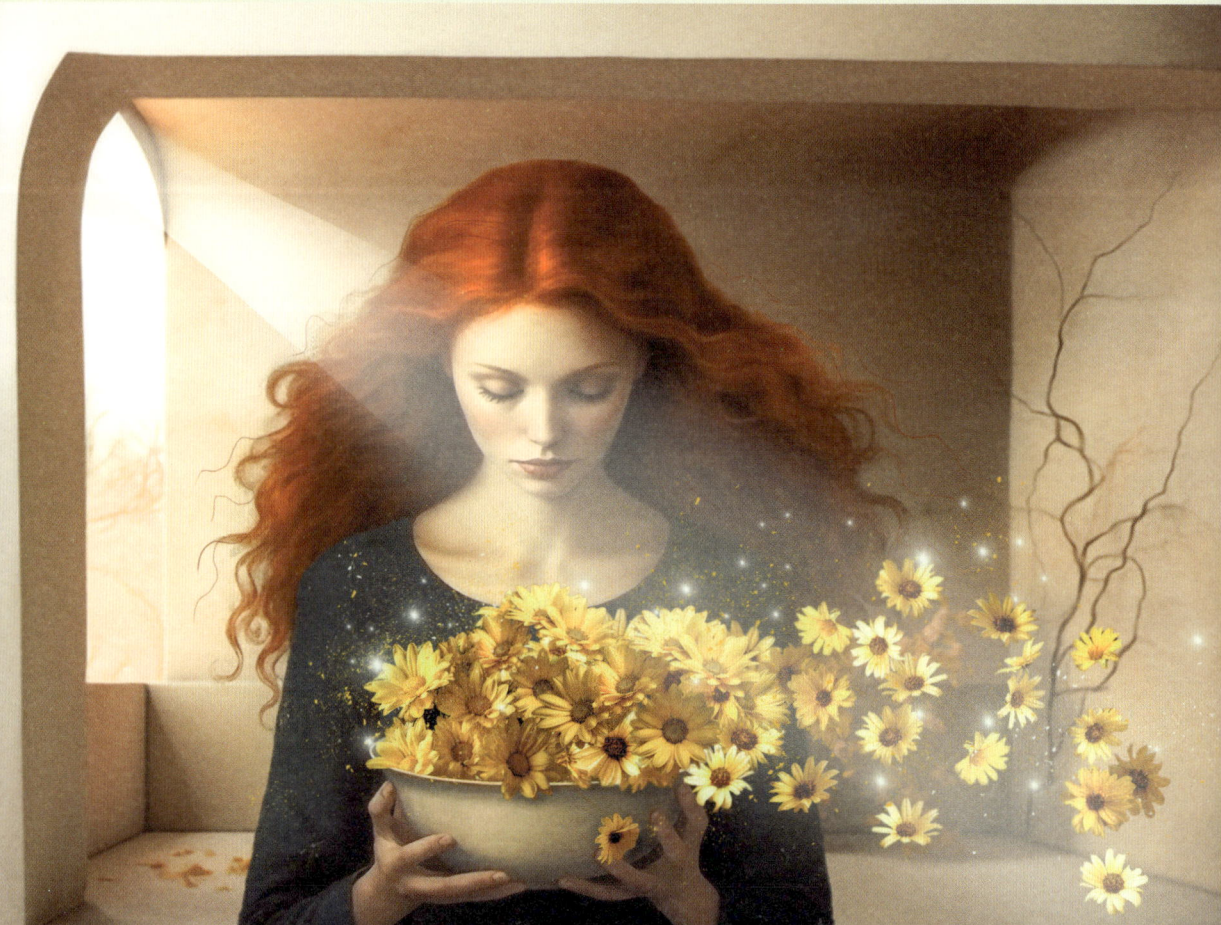

Sunchoke Soup
with Hazelnut Crumble

YOU WILL NEED:

- 2 crushed garlic cloves
- 1 onion, finely diced
- 17 ounces (500 g) of peeled and cubed sunchoke
- 4 cups (1 l) of vegetable broth
- 1/2 cup (100 ml) of coconut milk
- 1.7 ounces (50 g) of toasted and chopped hazelnuts
- Extra virgin olive oil
- Salt and pepper to taste

In a large pot, heat a drizzle of extra virgin olive oil and add garlic and onion. Sauté over medium heat until they become translucent. Add the sunchoke cubes and stir well to season. Cook for about five minutes. Pour the vegetable broth into the pot and bring to a boil. Then reduce the heat and let it cook over medium-low heat for about twenty minutes, or until the sunchokes become soft, then blend the soup with an immersion blender until it takes on a creamy consistency. Now you can add the coconut milk and adjust the salt and pepper to taste, continuing to stir and cook for another five minutes. Remove from the heat, serve in bowls, and garnish with the chopped hazelnuts.

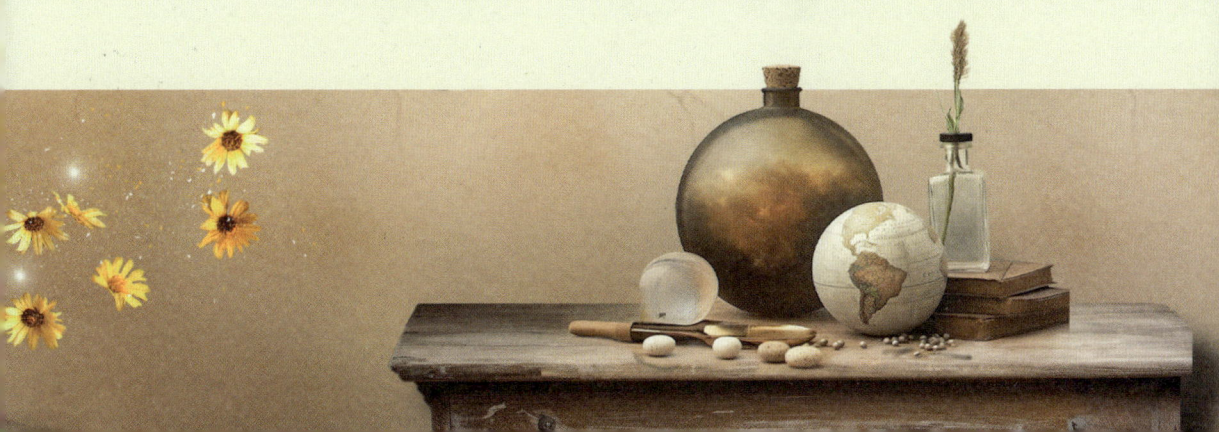

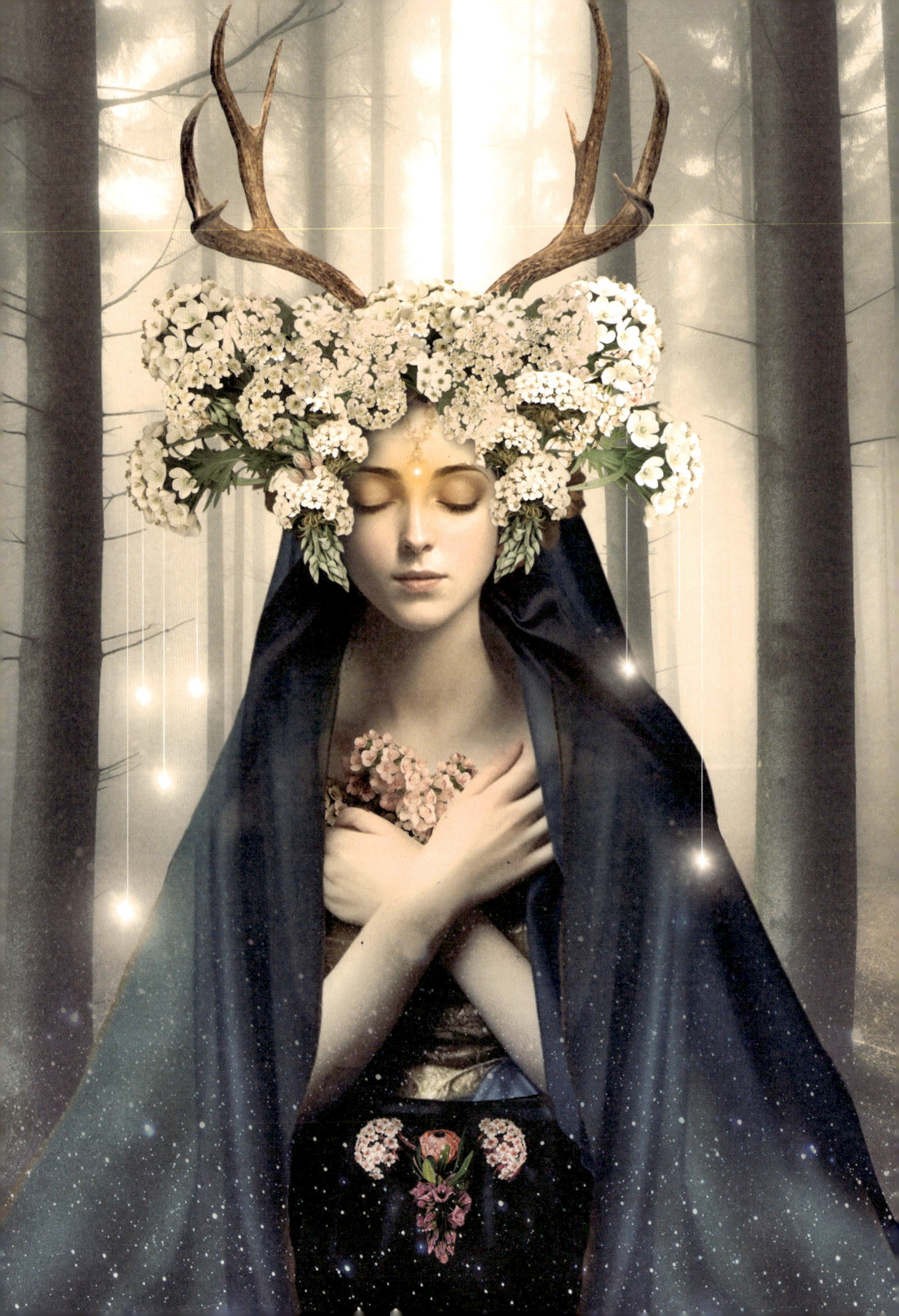

YARROW

— ACHILLEA MILLEFOLIUM —

Yarrow is an herbaceous plant recognizable by its distinctive leaves, which appear to be composed of other tiny leaflets: hence the name, *millefolium*. The small white flowers are grouped in flat, round inflorescences. It is a common plant in many regions of the world because of its ability to adapt to different soils and climatic conditions. The name *Achillea* comes from the myth of Achilles. It is said that the plant, known for its healing properties, was the secret to his invincibility. From a phytotherapeutic point of view, in fact, it has excellent healing properties. Application of an infusion or oil made from yarrow can accelerate the formation of scar tissue and protect the skin from infection. It also has good hemostatic properties, which means it helps stop bleeding; in the past, it was used in first aid on small wounds. The plant is also useful for regulating the menstrual cycle and can be taken as an herbal tea.

– MAGICAL USES –

In magic, yarrow repels negative energy, acting on the person's ability to create healthy boundaries. The plant is associated with personal protection, particularly the development of our ability to say no and preserve vital space. It acts positively on the ability to be alone and enjoy fruitful solitude. In addition, yarrow is often used in divination rituals and spells related to wisdom and vision. Its dried leaves can be burned as incense to foster spiritual connection and mental clarity during magical practices. In I Ching divination, yarrow stems were used before coins. Based on how they were thrown and what pattern they formed as they fell, the corresponding hexagram was read.

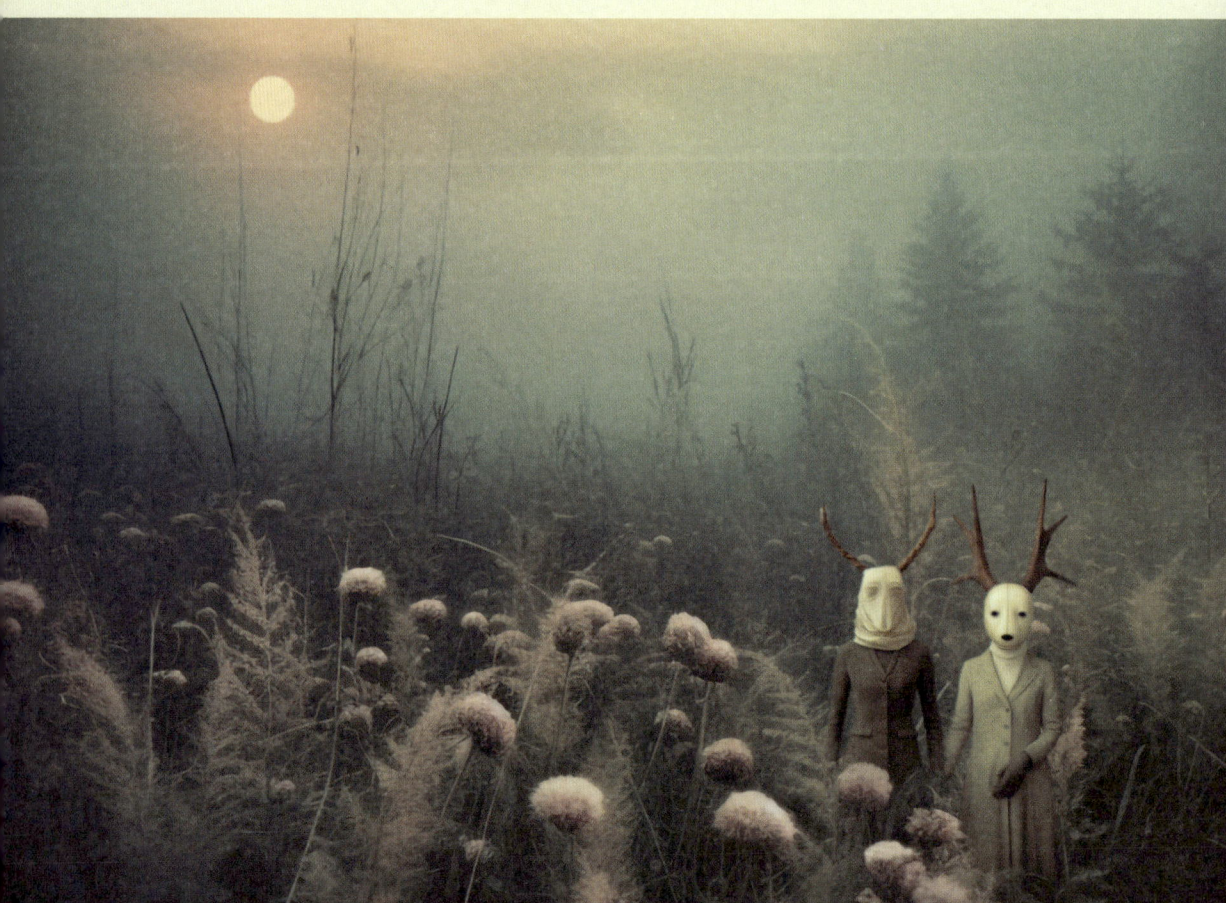

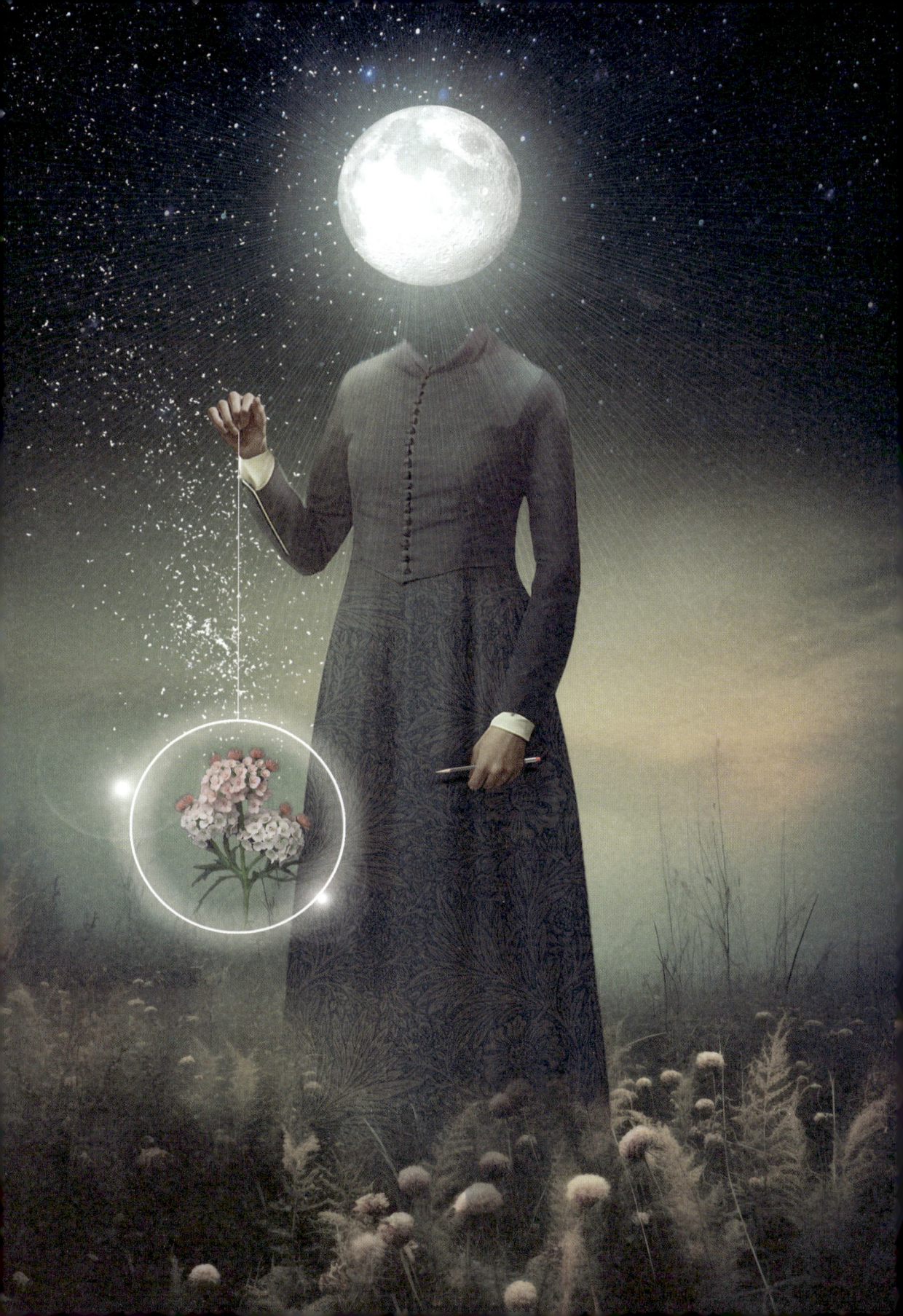

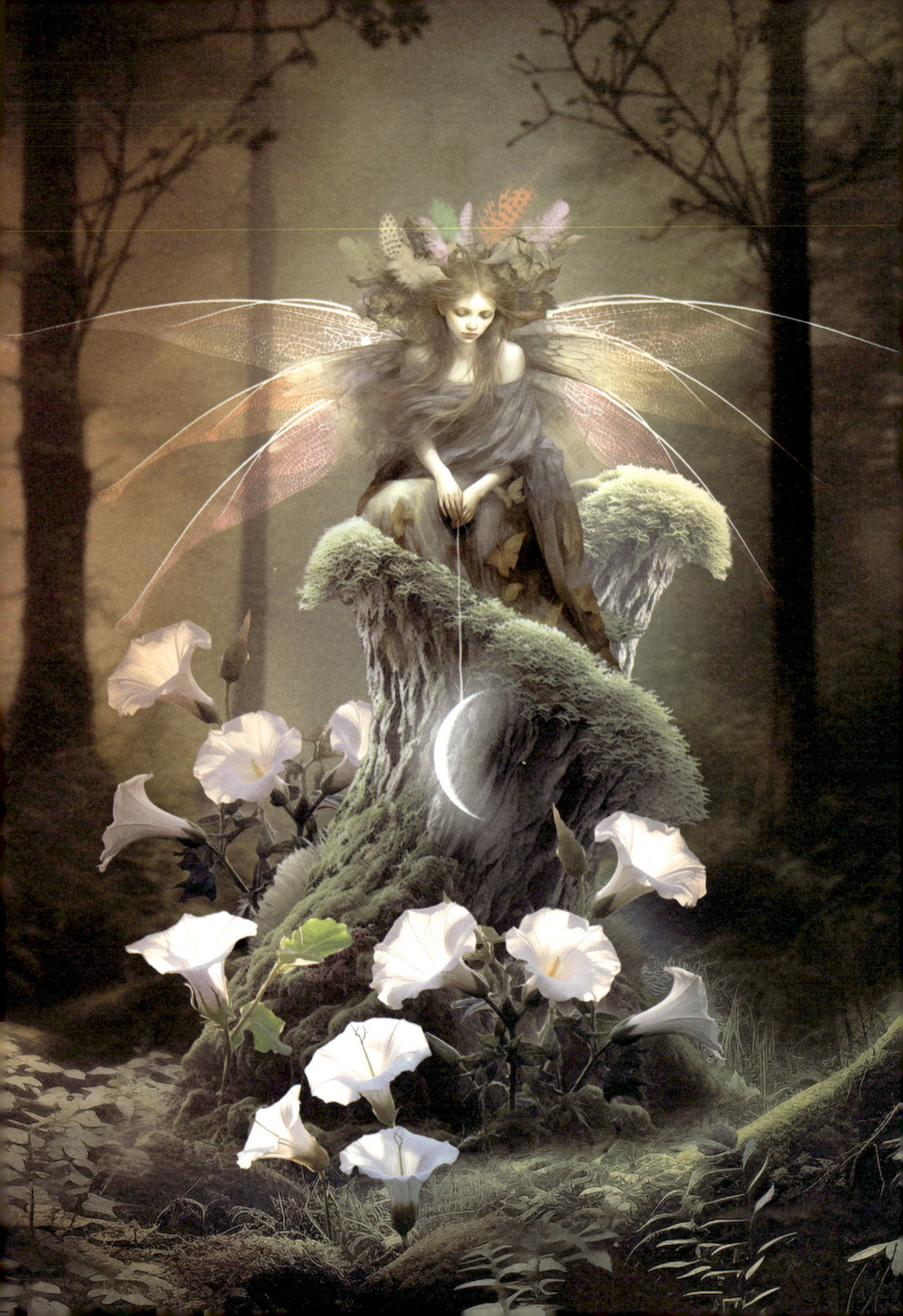

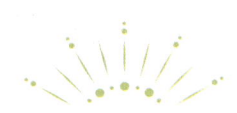

MORNING GLORY

— CONVOLVULUS ARVENSIS —

Just by looking at morning glory, the mind is immediately plunged into the world of fantasy. It is no coincidence that the Brothers Grimm included it in one of their fairy tales, *Our Lady's Little Glass*, as a cup from which a fairy drinks. Its flowers look like tiny goblets. Botanically speaking, it belongs to the Convolvulaceae family and is distinguished by its heart-shaped leaves, slender vines, and trumpet-shaped flowers, often white in color, that open at first light and close again in the evening, hence its common name. In the past, the plant was used for its laxative effects, but it is always good to act with great caution, as some bindweed species are poisonous; internal use is stronglydiscouraged. In ancient times, this plant was believed to be inhabited by spirits and fairy creatures. Its bell-shaped flowers were said to have the power to attract love to those who wore them, and the flowers were the chalices of fairies, from which they drank the morning dew.

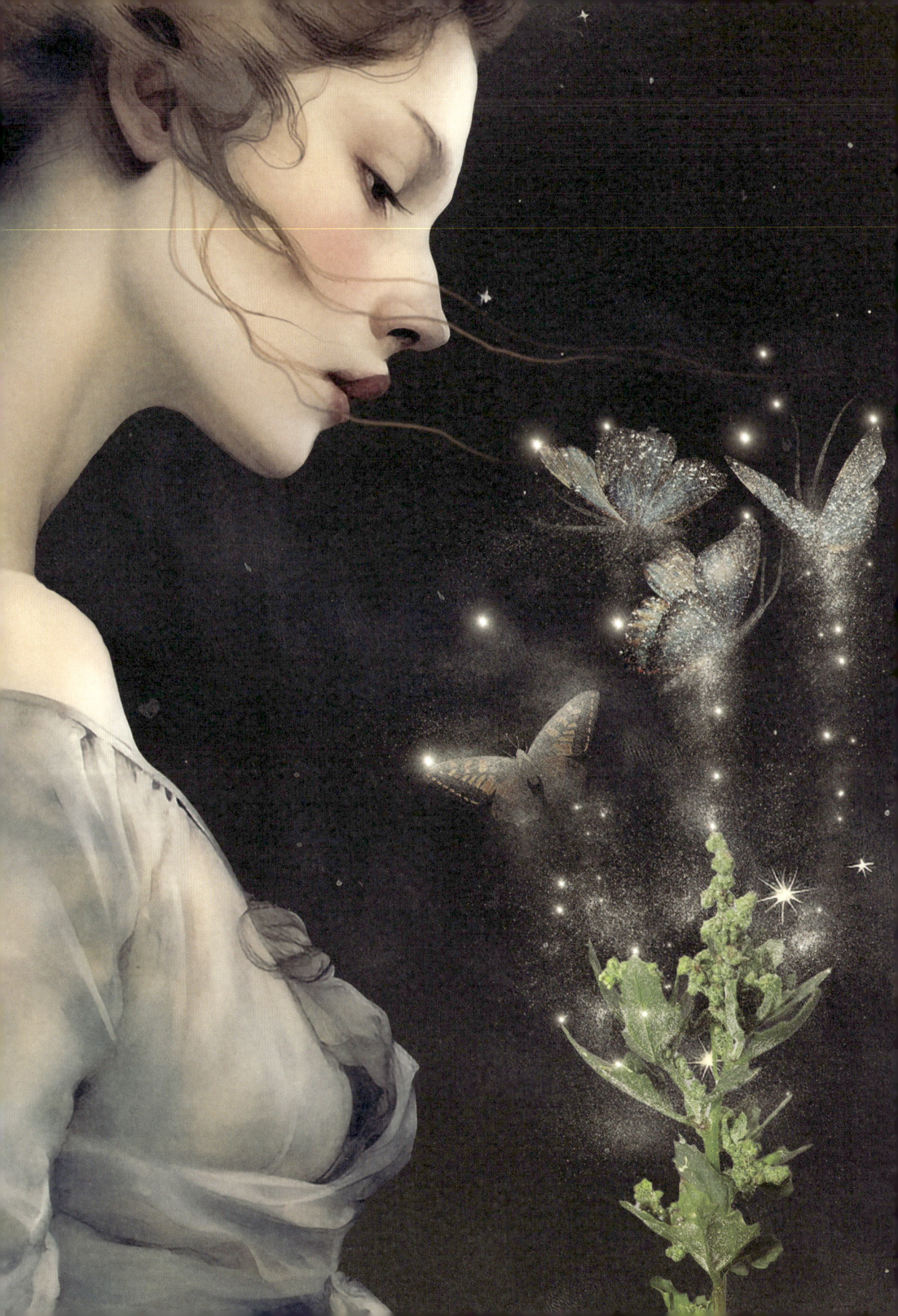

WILD SPINACH

— CHENOPODIUM ALBUM —

Wild spinach belongs to the Chenopodiaceae family and is characterized by green leaves sprinkled with a fluffy white powder, a protective fuzz that gives the plant a distinctive appearance. The young, tender leaves can be used in cooking to enrich salads, soups, or savory pies and give them a tart, herbaceous touch. But they can also be used for their astringent, diuretic, and anti-inflammatory properties. Because of these properties, the plant can be used to relieve gastrointestinal disorders. The leaves are rich in nutrients such as vitamins (A, C, K) and minerals (calcium, iron, potassium), and thus help strengthen the immune system and overall health of the body. From an energy point of view, wild spinach is related to the simplicity of life, the appreciation of small daily pleasures. Its simplicity helps remind us of our own simplicity.

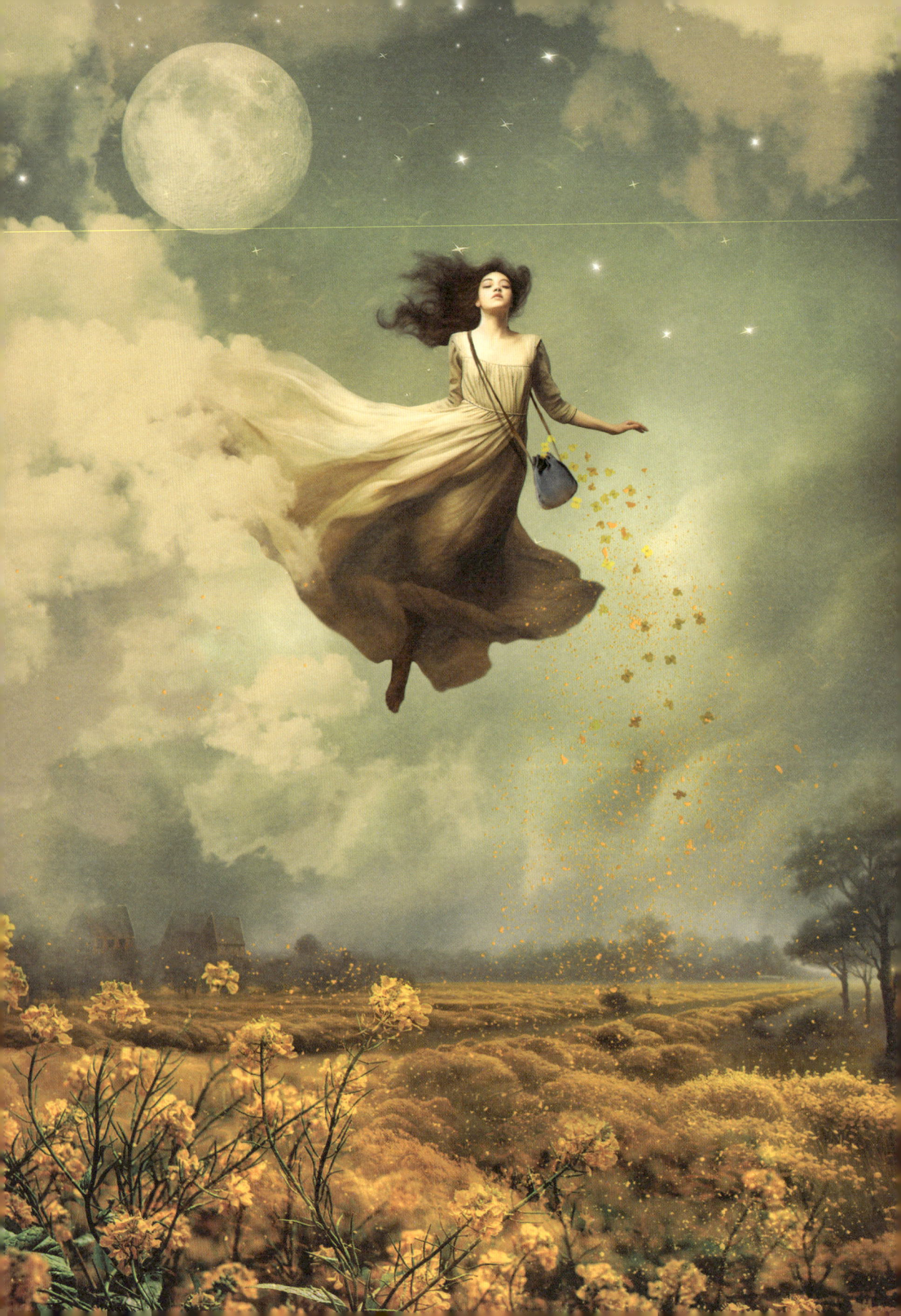

WILD MUSTARD

— Sinapis arvensis —

Wild mustard, also called charlock, is easily recognized. It can reach a height of 3 feet (1 meter) and has dark green leaves with jagged edges and a lanceolate shape. The flowers are small, bright yellow, and they're clustered in inflorescences that develop along the stems. The seeds, which are round and contained in small pods called siliques, when ripe, are harvested and used to make mustard powder or for the production of mustard oil. From an herbalist perspective, the seeds have analgesic, antibiotic, and anti-inflammatory characteristics. There are ancient remedies that involve making compresses with the ground seeds and water, and then placing them on the chest of someone with a cough, or inhaling the vapors given off by the seeds to clear the nose in cases of congestion. It is a plant connected to Mars, given its fire sign and pungency. It was widespread in rural Italy, where seeds were scattered before the front door to keep out negative energy.

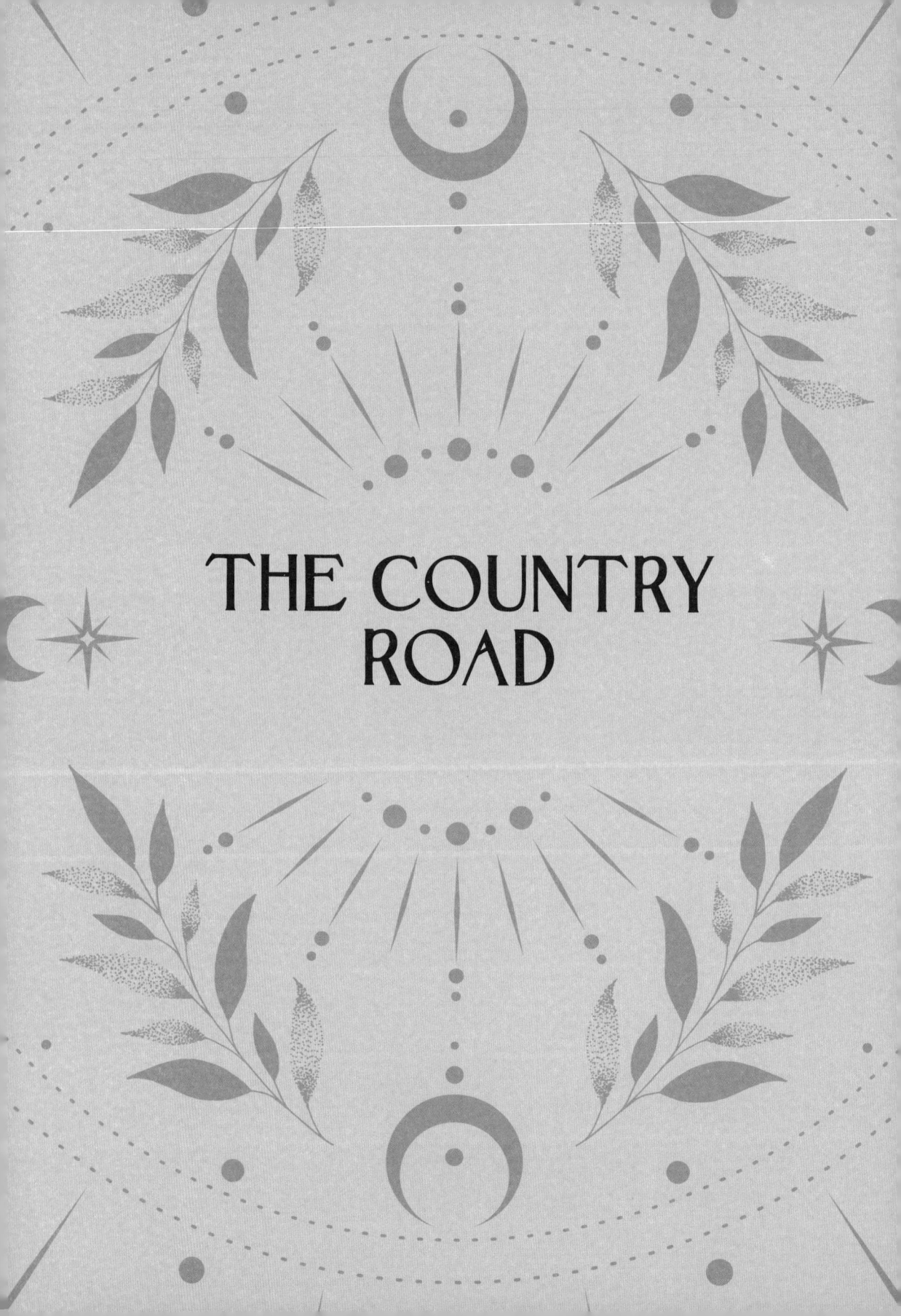

THE COUNTRY
ROAD

Outside every village there is a road that winds like a shiny ribbon across the countryside. You can take it at any hour of the day or night, but the most magical moment is at dusk, when the light turns golden and the first stars begin to shine in the indigo sky. There is a moment when heaven and Earth seem to merge, when boundaries disappear and we are immersed in the whole. Only at that moment do you begin to grasp everything around you with full consciousness. The grasses by the side of the path seem to dance in the evening air, and if you brush your fingers over the spearmint growing nearby you will carry its scent with you into the night. Crickets play their evening symphony and accompany the distant hooting of an owl, barely awake in the twilight. The air is filled with intense, earthy scents, the smell of wet earth mingling with the sweet aroma of nighttime flowers. Each flower is a small explosion of color, like the fireworks at village festivals in midsummer. Along this road, which opens the soul to wonder, one may come across an isolated house with a gate covered in ivy, concealing its mystery from the eyes of travelers. This is the house of the rural witch. This witch holds all the wisdom of the countryside in the endless dance of nature's cycles, in the plants that grow luxuriantly, in the secrets guarded by the fertile soil, and she pours it into her remedies, syrups, and jars filled with herbs and roots. The country witch, with her piercing gaze and wise hands, is the living link between humanity and the ancient wisdom of the Earth. The country road beckons, inviting you to enter a wilder land, following the song of nocturnal insects, pausing for a moment in the violet breath of the sky, just before the moon rises.

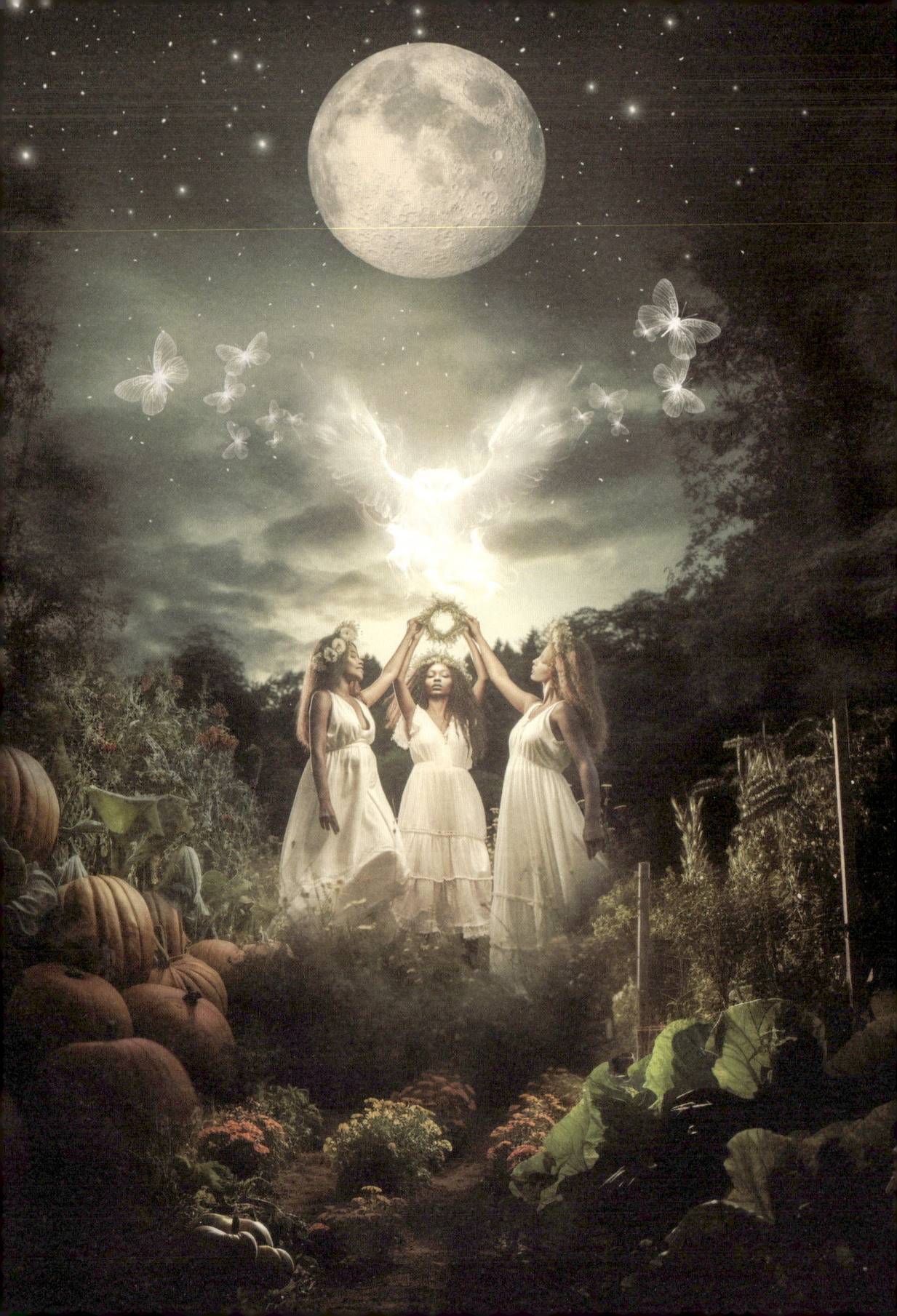

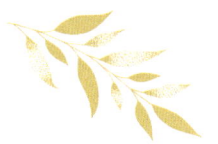
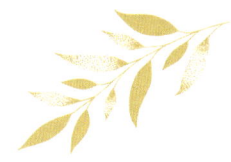

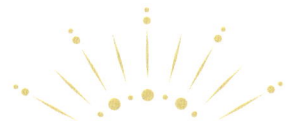

THE RURAL
WITCH

—

The imagery conjured by the rural
witch dates back to ancient times,
when knowledge of herbs and natural
remedies was fundamental to the
survival of rural communities.

Rural witches were considered custodians of ancestral wisdom, ancient healing, and divination practices passed down from generation to generation. Through their profound knowledge of plant properties, rituals, and moon phases, they can cure illnesses, relieve pain, and increase people's well-being.

Folktales are full of stories of rural witches who would gather in the woods, dance under the moonlight, and prepare magical potions.

It was believed that these women could change form and communicate with animal spirits, transcending the boundaries of the material world. In particular, the rural witch is an expert on herbs. Whether wild or cultivated, medicinal or edible, she can recognize them and knows where to forage them. She is aware of the richness of everything around us.

The rural witch often has a vegetable garden, and it, too, has a magical appeal. It allows her to connect with the magic of the little things that grow and have their own life cycle.

Like the Queen of Pentacles in a tarot deck, this witch is always welcoming and can heal the sick by appealing to folk practices. For example, for rural witches in the mountains of Tuscany, a common practice was to "remove fear" with *Stachys recta*, known as "witch weed" in Italian. The wild plant was used in various folk traditions for its calming properties that can alleviate fear and anxiety. The practice is done by preparing an infusion with the leaves or flowers of *Stachys recta*. The leaves and flowers are placed in a pot with water and brought to a boil, and, once the infusion has cooled, it is used to wash people who wish to "remove fear."

> The knowledge of the rural witch, however, goes beyond herbalist practices. It is subtle and stems from her ability to listen to plants. Plants are her friends, and the garden is her chosen place for enchantments and magic.

You can see her tying copper bells to tomatoes to make them grow better, or having tea with the lilies of the valley that grow by the door of her house. Her special power is simplicity. She waits for you, sitting on the step of her house, a cup of lemon balm infusion in her hands, lulled by the song of crickets, grateful for the abundance of life.

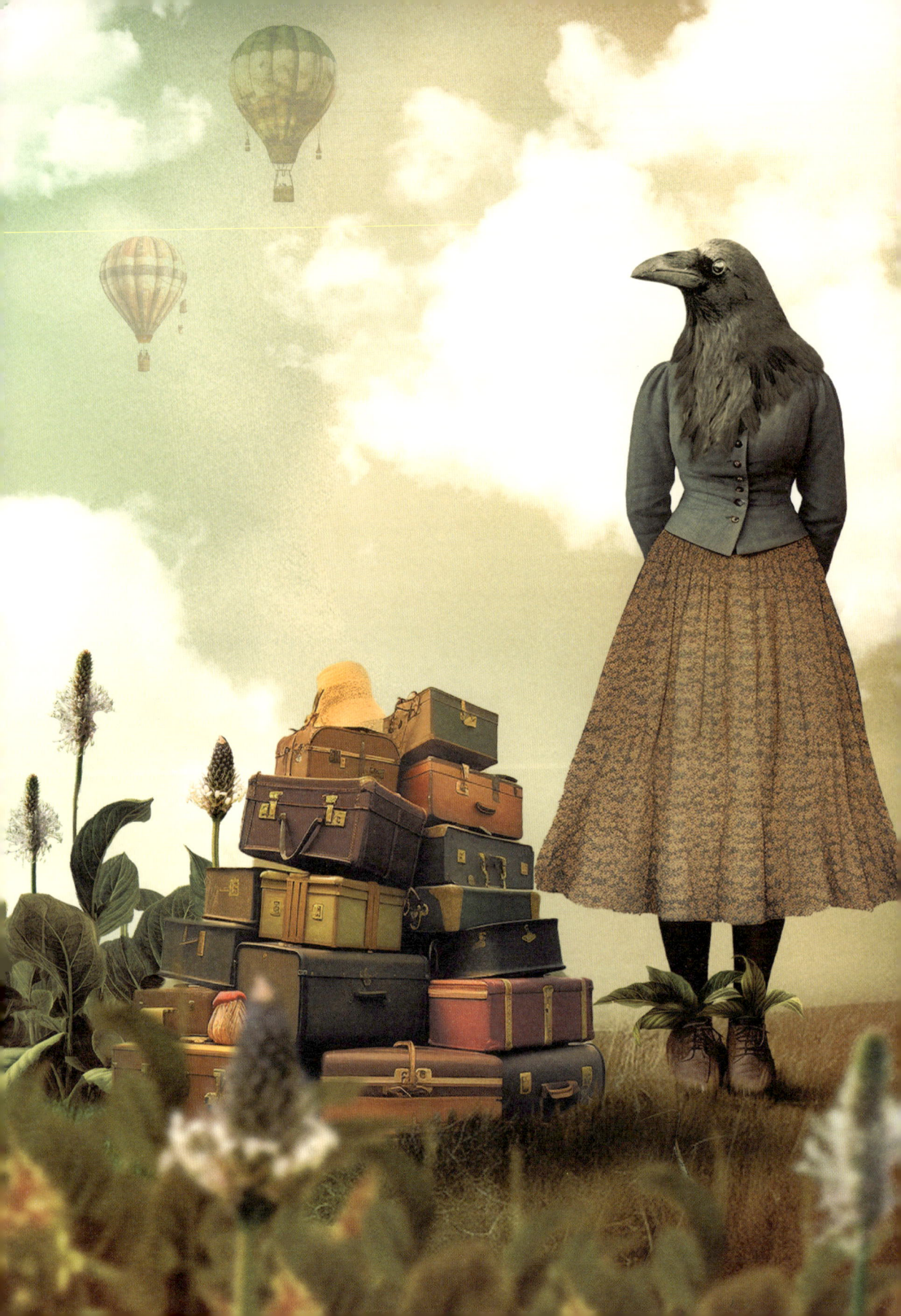

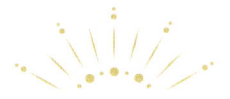

BROADLEAF PLANTAIN

– Plantago major
or Plantago lanceolata –

Broadleaf plantain is often found near houses. In phytotherapy, it is valued for its anti-inflammatory and soothing properties. Its leaves, rich in mucilage, can be used to soothe inflammation of the respiratory system. An infusion of its leaves can be a natural remedy for sore throats and coughs, while syrup prepared from its leaves helps with oily coughs because of its mucolytic effect. In ancient times, the plant was associated with snakes; because of its protective power, it was thought to expel venom from the body. Although this is not the case, the plant retains protective and purifying characteristics, albeit on a subtle level. It is said that putting a plantain leaf in shoes will protect a traveler on the road.

– CULINARY USES –

Plantain is an excellent food. Its young leaves can be harvested and added to salads, offering a touch of freshness and a wide variety of nutrients such as vitamins A, C, and K as well as potassium and calcium. There are several species of plantain, the most common being Plantago major (major plantain) and Plantago lanceolata (minor plantain). Both species exhibit similar character-istics, but major has larger and wider leaves than minor, which has longer, semi-erect ones. For food use, you can harvest the leaves or the seeds, which appear after flowering on the spikes. It is nicknamed poor man's asparagus and can be used to flavor many dishes.

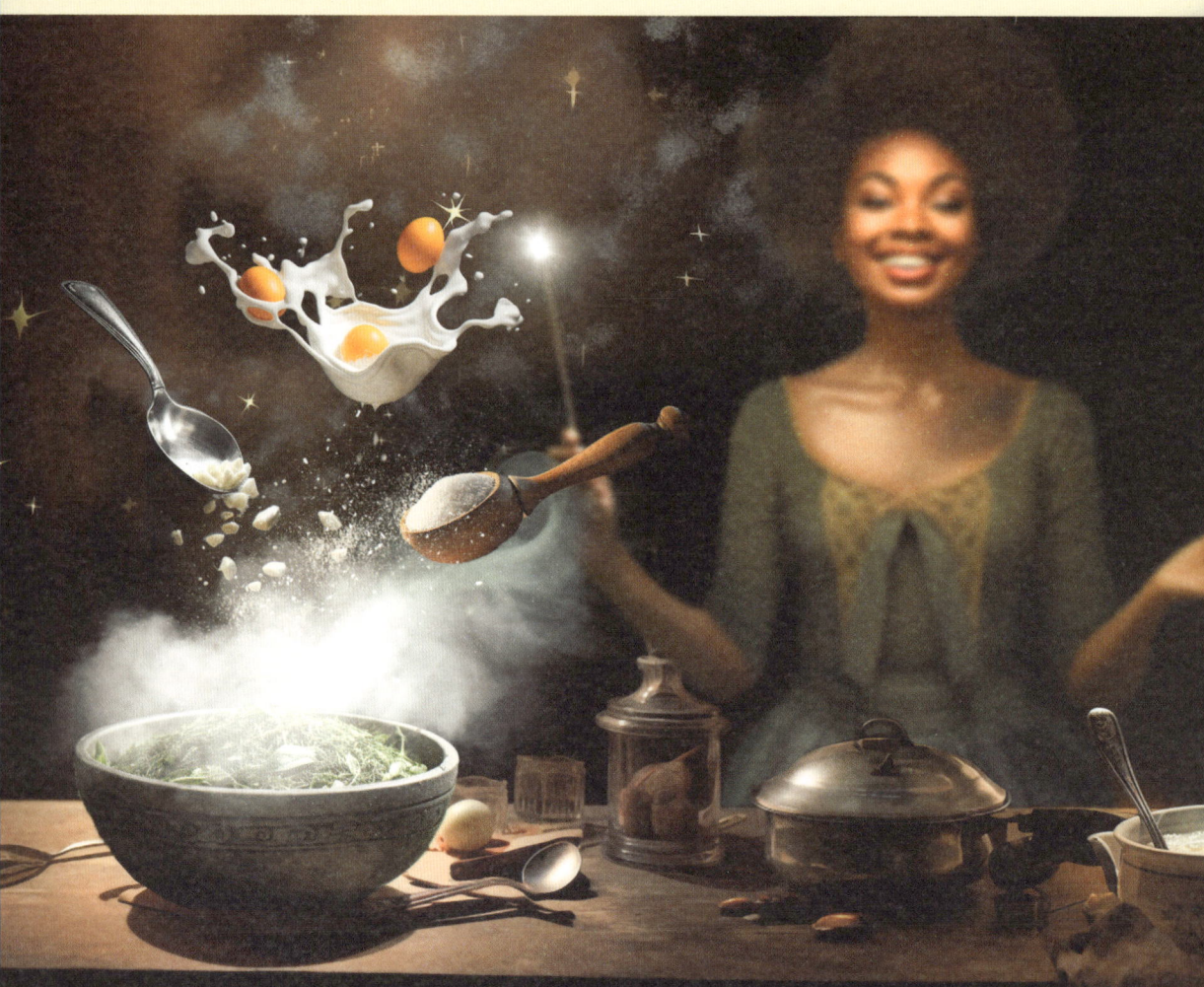

Broadleaf Plantain Flan

YOU WILL NEED:

- 2 bunches of plantain leaves
- 5 or 6 white potatoes
- 2 eggs or 4 spoonfuls of chickpea flour
- 1/2 cup (100 ml) of soy milk
- 1.7 ounces (50 g) of grated cheese (parmesan or pecorino) or nutritional yeast for vegans
- Salt and pepper to taste
- Olive oil to grease the pan

Heat the oven to 350°F (180°C) and grease a baking sheet with olive oil. Boil the potatoes, peeled and cut into pieces, and blanch the plantain leaves for four to five minutes in boiling salted water. In a bowl, beat the eggs with the milk, then add the grated cheese. When the potatoes are boiled, mash them with a fork and add the chopped plantain leaves. Mix in the vegetables, add salt and pepper, and bake for twenty-five to thirty minutes.

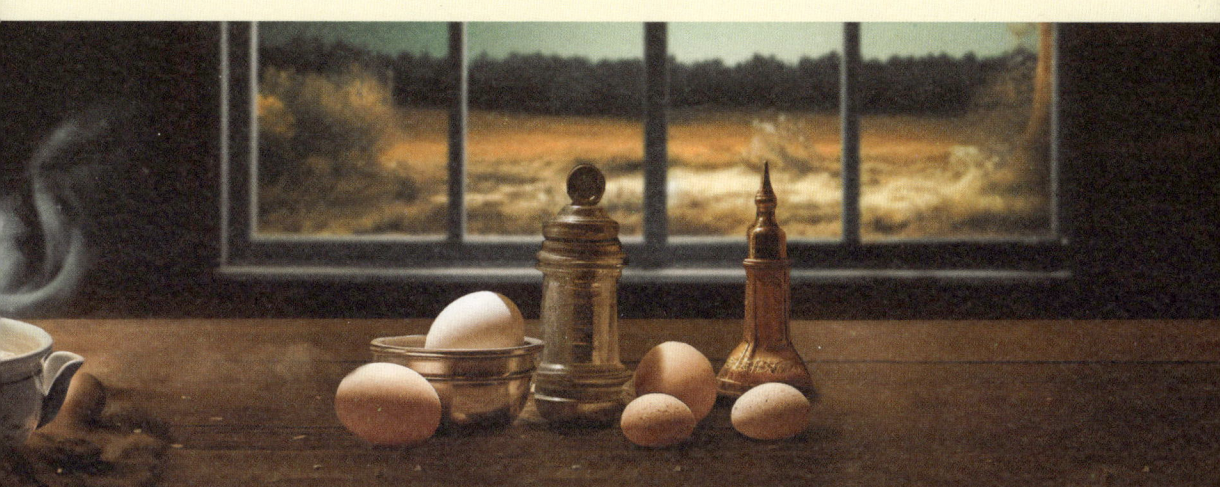

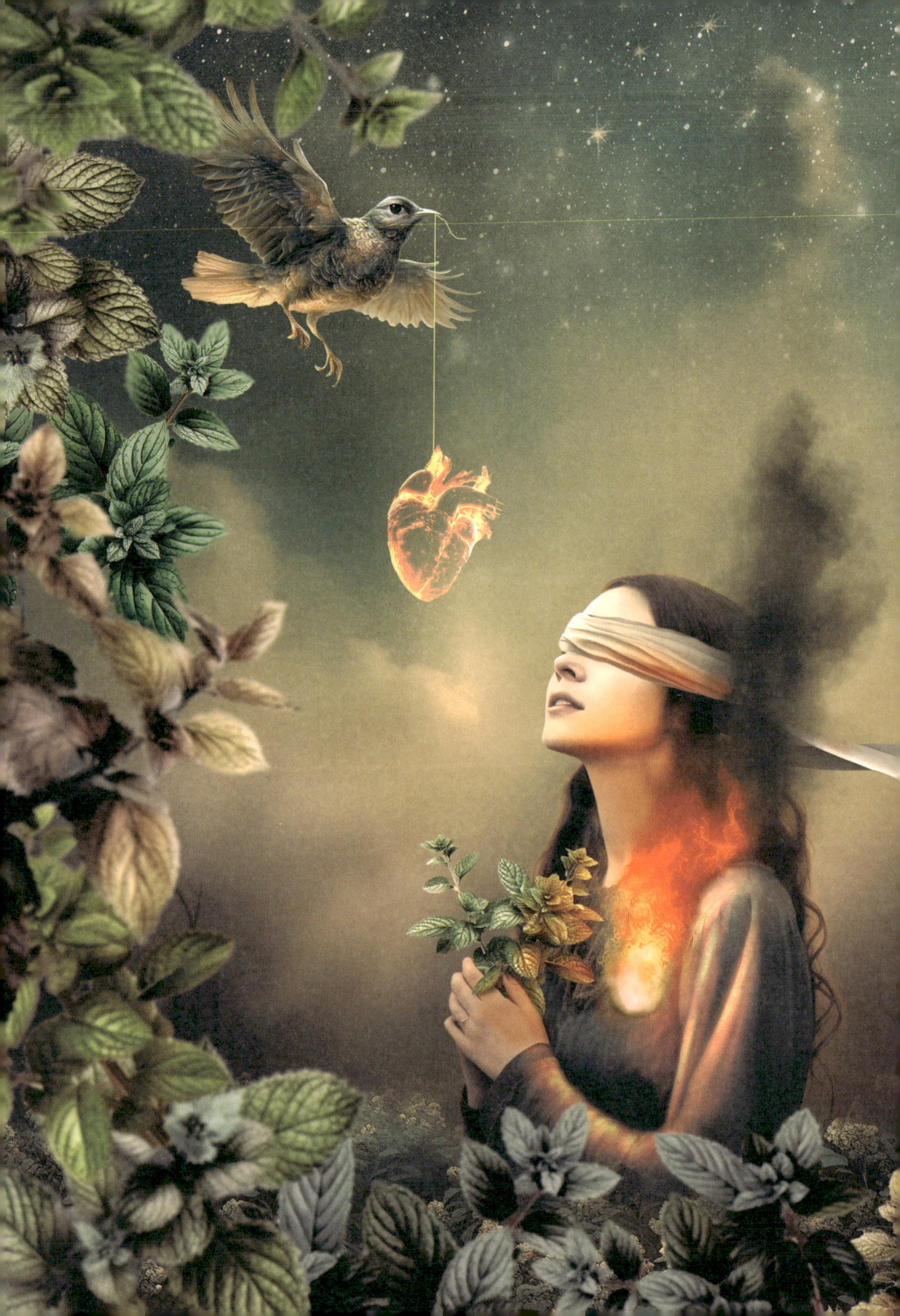

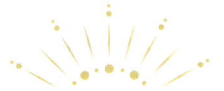

WILD MINT

— Mentha arvensis —

Mint is a very communicative plant. As soon as you enter a field it inhabits, even before you see it, you can identify it by its scent. In phytotherapy, it is famous for its digestive and carminative properties. Its essential oil contains menthol, which helps relax the muscles of the digestive system, thus relieving spasms and abdominal pain. An infusion of its leaves can be used to relieve ailments such as indigestion, abdominal bloating, and nausea. Mint is also valued for its calming properties—inhaling or applying mint essential oil to the skin can help reduce tension— and for its cooling effect on the body, especially in summer. It provides relief to tired legs, and is useful as an after-sun treatment. It is a valuable companion in meditation. Its scent can aid concentration and, when used in divination rituals, promote understanding of hidden messages in the universe.

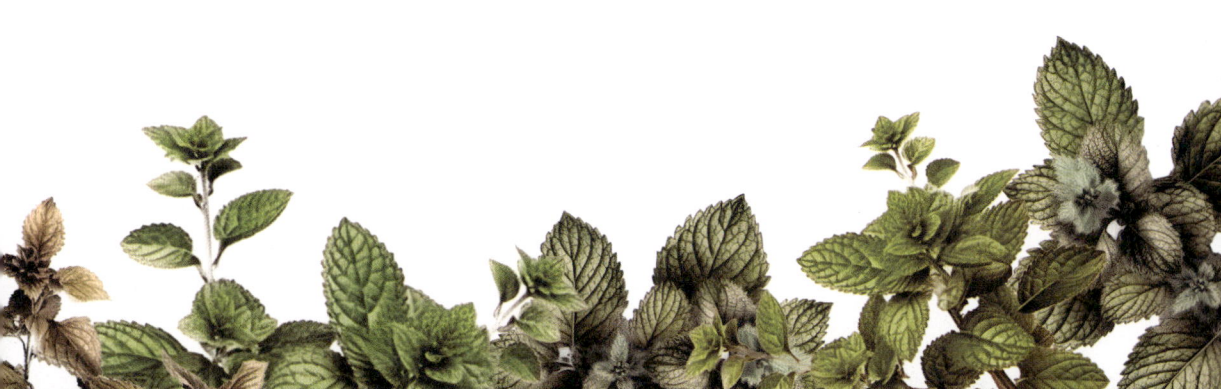

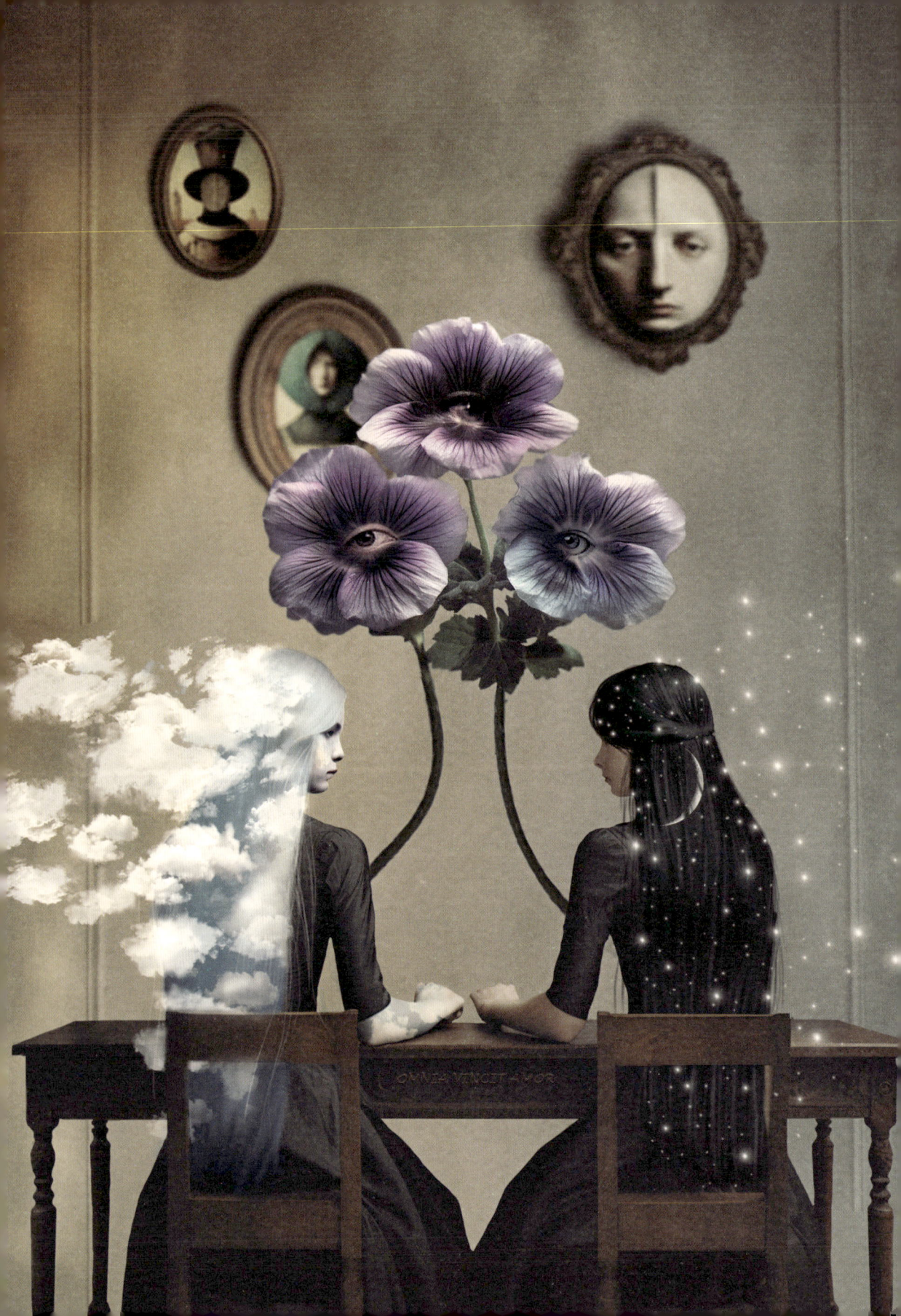

MALLOW

– Malva sylvestris –

The pink-and-green mallow peers out from the sides of country lanes with its soft, heart-shaped leaves. It is a delicate plant that speaks directly to the souls of those who are smaller: children, animals, elves, and fairies. Since ancient times, mallow has been widely used for its soothing, anti-inflammatory, and emollient properties. Leaves and flowers contain mucilage, a gelatinous substance that gives the plant a velvety texture and can protect mucous membranes against irritation, for example in the respiratory system. Mallow is often used to relieve skin irritations through compresses or infusions of its leaves. In folk tradition, mallow is associated with love and divination. Its petals were used in love spells, whereas the leaves enhanced intuition and psychic perception. It was said to bring harmony to relationships and promote loving communication.

– COSMETIC USES –

Mallow, with its delicate beauty and beneficial properties, is an ally in skin and hair care. Thanks to its emollient properties, it is particularly suitable for soothing and moisturizing dry, sensitive, or irritated skin. It can be used in the preparation of creams, lotions, and balms for the body, helping to relieve itching, redness, and inflammation. It can also be used for oral care by making an infusion of its leaves and flowers as a mouthwash.

Mallow Hydrating Lotion

YOU WILL NEED:

- 1 cup of distilled water
- 1 cup of mallow flowers and leaves
- 2 spoonfuls of vegetable glycerin
- 2 spoonfuls of coconut oil
- 1 spoonful of shea butter
- 1 spoonful of beeswax
- 10 drops of lavender essential oil (optional)

In a pot, bring the distilled water to a boil. Add the mallow leaves and flowers, then let the pot boil for about 10 minutes. This will help extract the mucilage and other beneficial active ingredients. After ten minutes, remove the pot from the heat and let it cool slightly. Strain the mallow infusion. In another pot, melt the coconut oil, shea butter, and beeswax in a double boiler over low heat. Stir until smooth. Add the infusion to this oil mixture, and mix well. Let it cool and add the glycerin and the drops of essential oil. Pour the lotion into an airtight jar. Use it within two or three weeks.

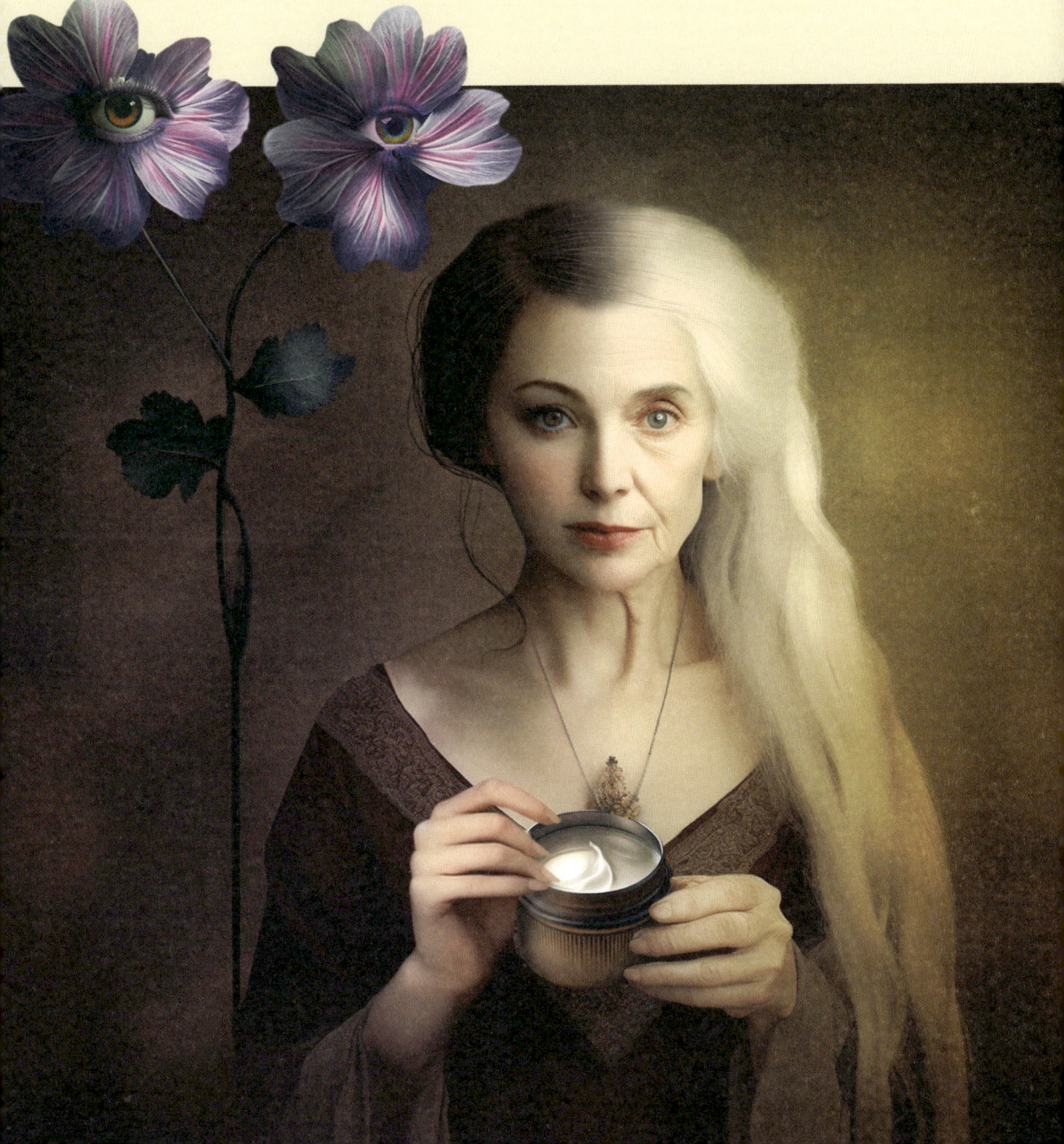

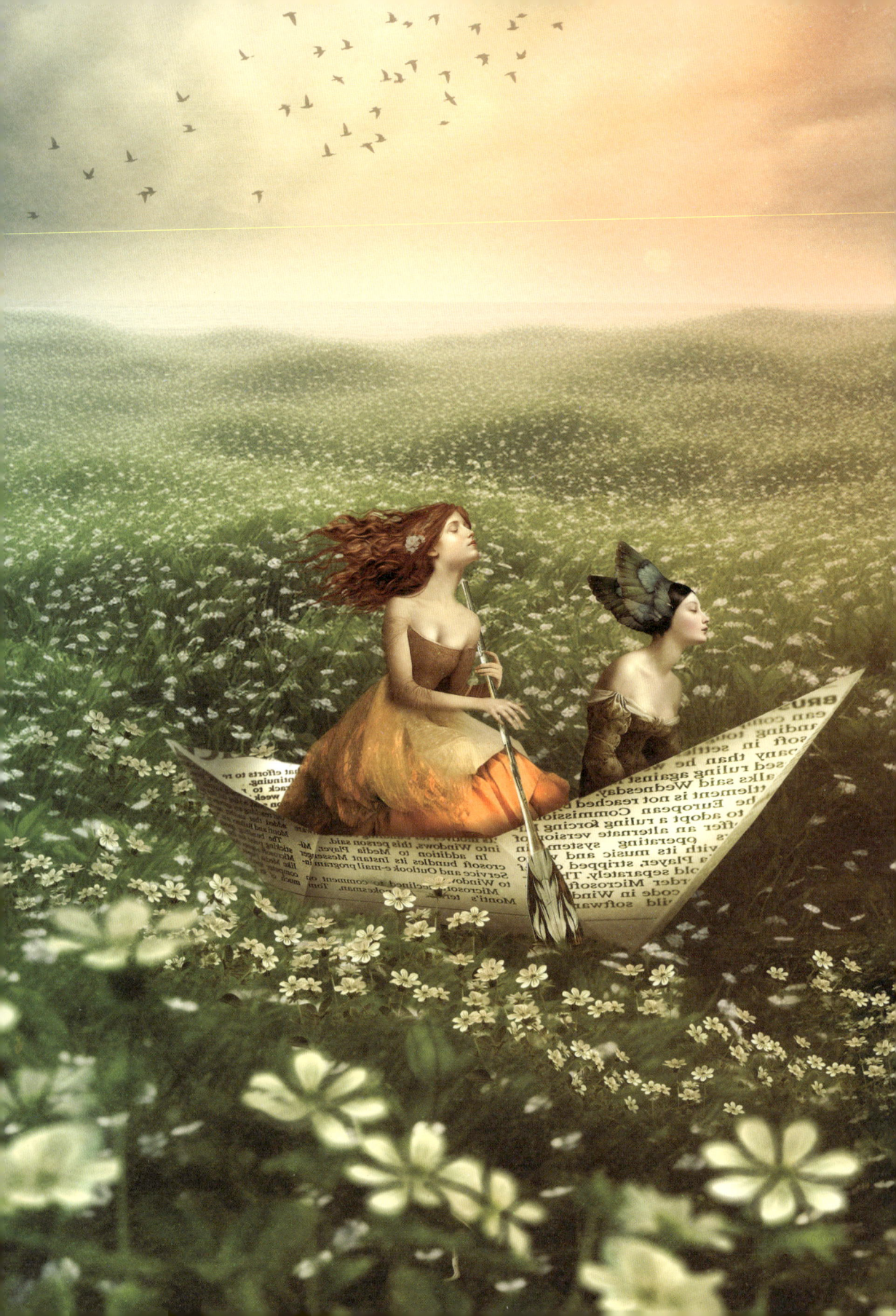

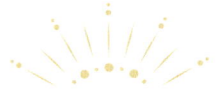

CHICKWEED

— Stellaria media —

Chickweed stares up from the country road with its tiny white flowers. When you come across it, as you surely have, it makes a field look like a green sky dotted with tiny stars. It is a fresh plant that can even grow in winter and can be eaten as an herb along with spinach and chard. In herbalism, its leaves and flowers contain beneficial substances such as flavonoids, saponins, and vitamin C, from which it derives its emollient and soothing properties. It can be used to relieve skin irritations, such as eczema and dermatitis, and to promote diuresis. According to tradition, chickweed is a bringer of good luck and protection. Hanging bouquets of chickweed above doorways or carrying them with you in a small bag is said to promote prosperity and ward off negative energy. It is connected to fidelity and love and brings harmony to relationships, fostering bonds in which true affection is nurtured.

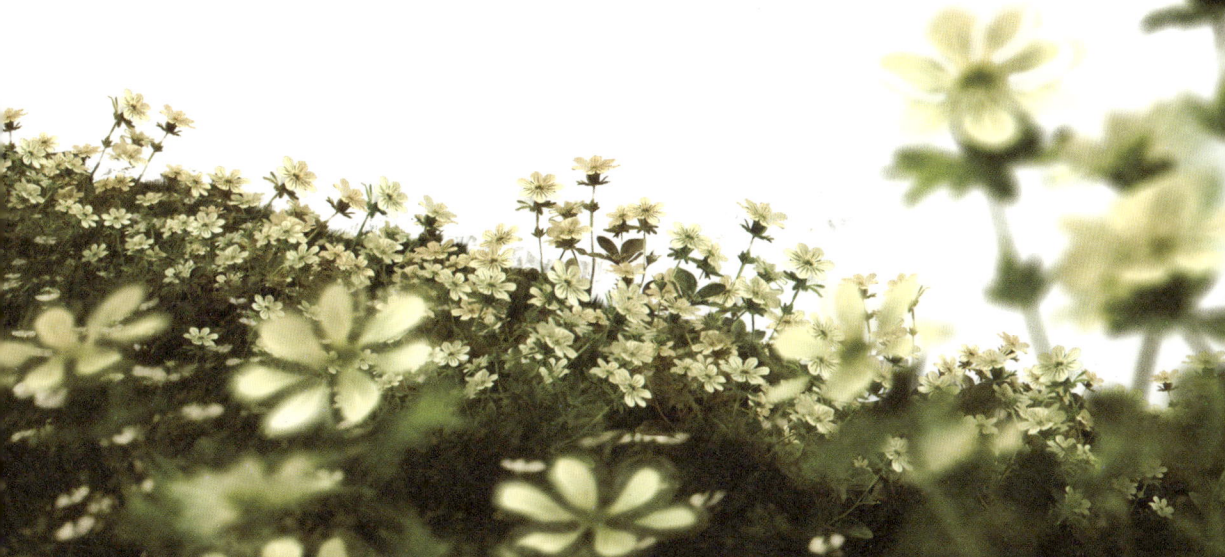

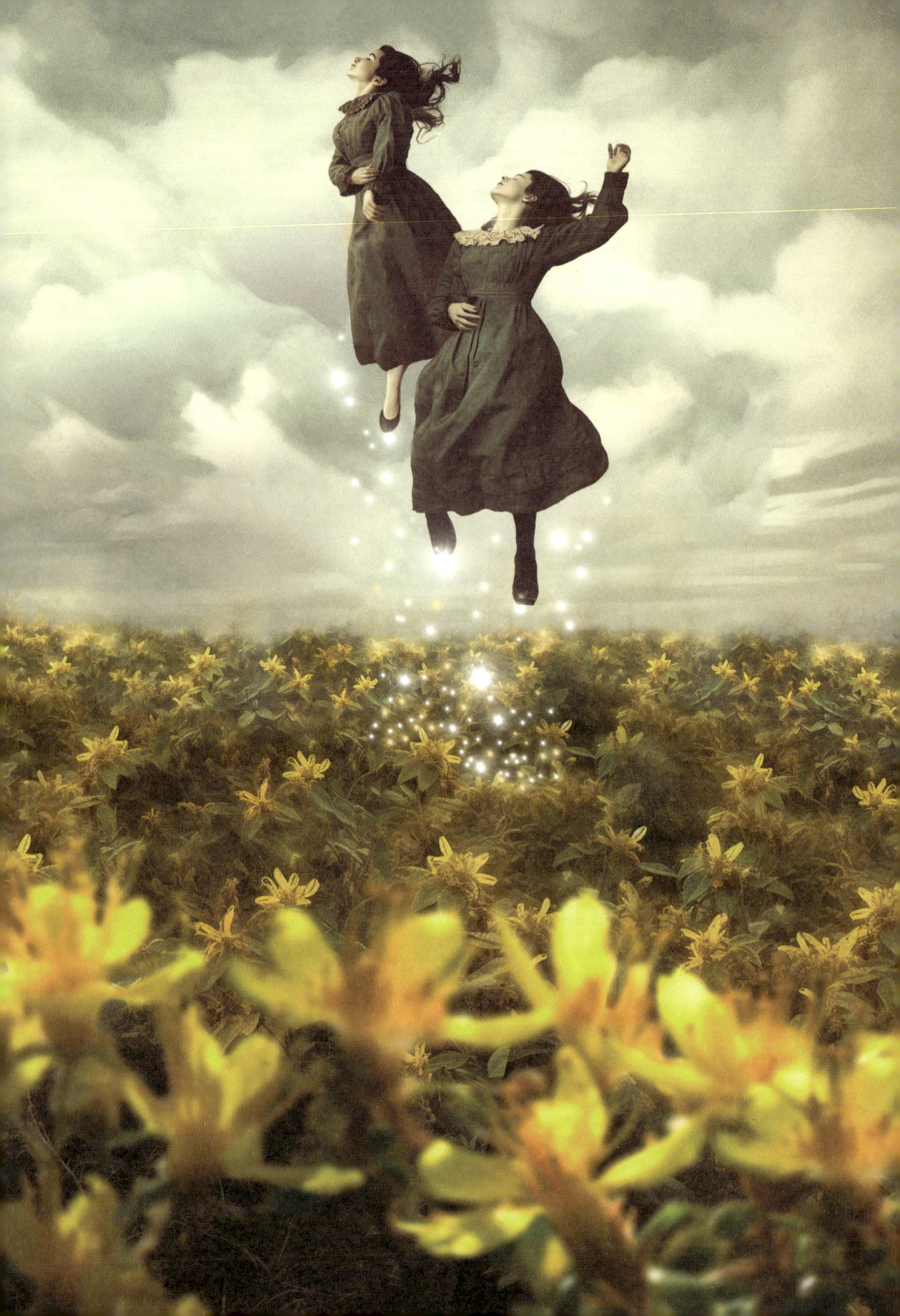

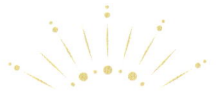

SAINT-JOHN'S-WORT

— HYPERICUM PERFORATUM —

The yellow star *Hypericum* shines on June evenings near the summer solstice. A magical plant par excellence, it carries the sign of the sun and summer. The name *perforatum* comes from its leaves containing resinous sacs, which, when viewed against light, look like small holes. The plant has great restorative abilities for small wounds, burns, or rashes. When taken, however, it acts as a natural antidepressant, as it interacts with serotonin reuptake, and can relieve anxiety and sleep disorders. The famous St. John's oil is prepared with the flowers, a bloodred oil that is an excellent remedy for rashes and can be used for invigorating massages, especially after sports.

Warning: it is important to point out that Saint-John's-wort is likely to interact with some medications, such as antidepressants, anticoagulants, and oral contraceptives. And it can also increase sun sensitivity, so the use of sunscreen is strongly recommended.

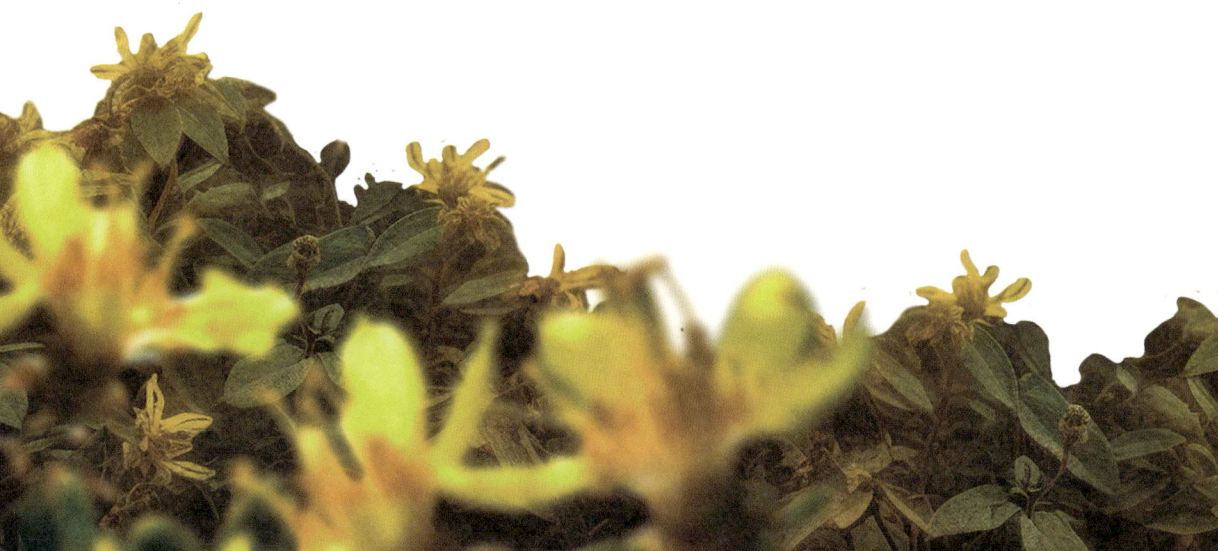

– MAGICAL USES –

You can harvest Saint-John's-wort in summer and use it for your enchantments. It is considered a very powerful magical plant, and legends and traditions date back to antiquity. It is associated with celebrations of St. John the Baptist, hence its common name. Saint-John's-wort is also said to have healing properties and can be used in amulets or talismans to bring good luck and protection. Hanging a bunch of Saint-John's-wort on your door, tied by a red thread, will ward off negativity until next summer.

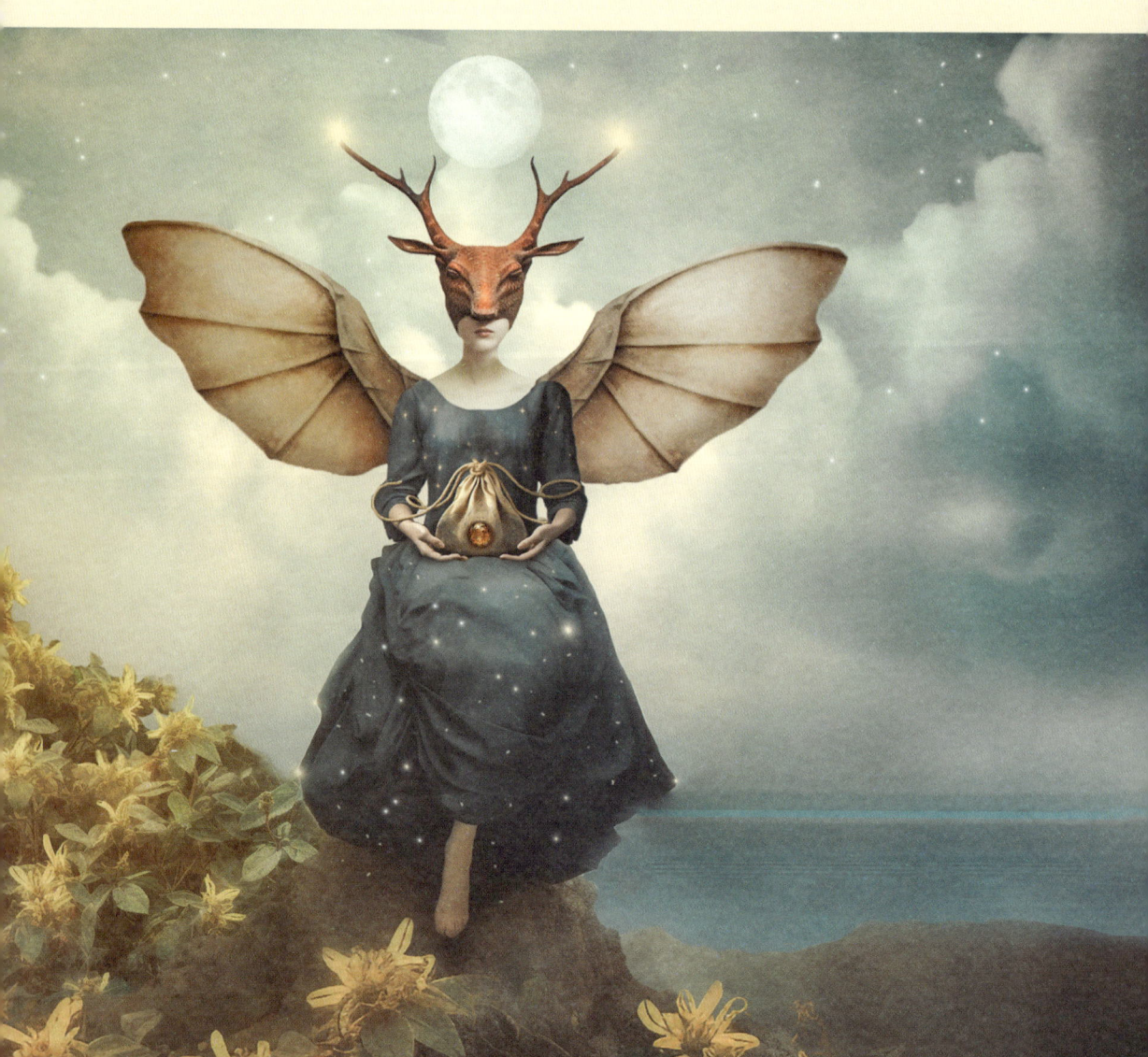

Summer Sachet

YOU WILL NEED:

- ❧ 1 small gold or yellow cloth bag
- ❧ 1 cup of dried Saint-John's-wort flowers
- ❧ 1 clear quartz crystal
- ❧ 3 drops of lavender essential oil
- ❧ 1 piece of gold ribbon

Take the small bag of gold or yellow cloth and hold it in your hands, focusing on your intention for healing and protection. Add the dried Saint-John's-wort flowers to the small bag. Visualize the golden light emanating from the Saint-John's-wort and add the clear quartz crystal to the small bag. This crystal will amplify the energy of Saint-John's-wort and help focus the intention of your magic. Add the drops of lavender essential oil. Lavender will bring calm and harmony, increasing the healing and protective effects of your sachet. Finally, close it off with a gold ribbon. While doing so, imagine that the ribbon seals the magical energy inside the bag, charging it with good vibrations.

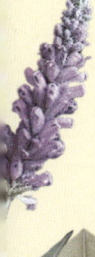

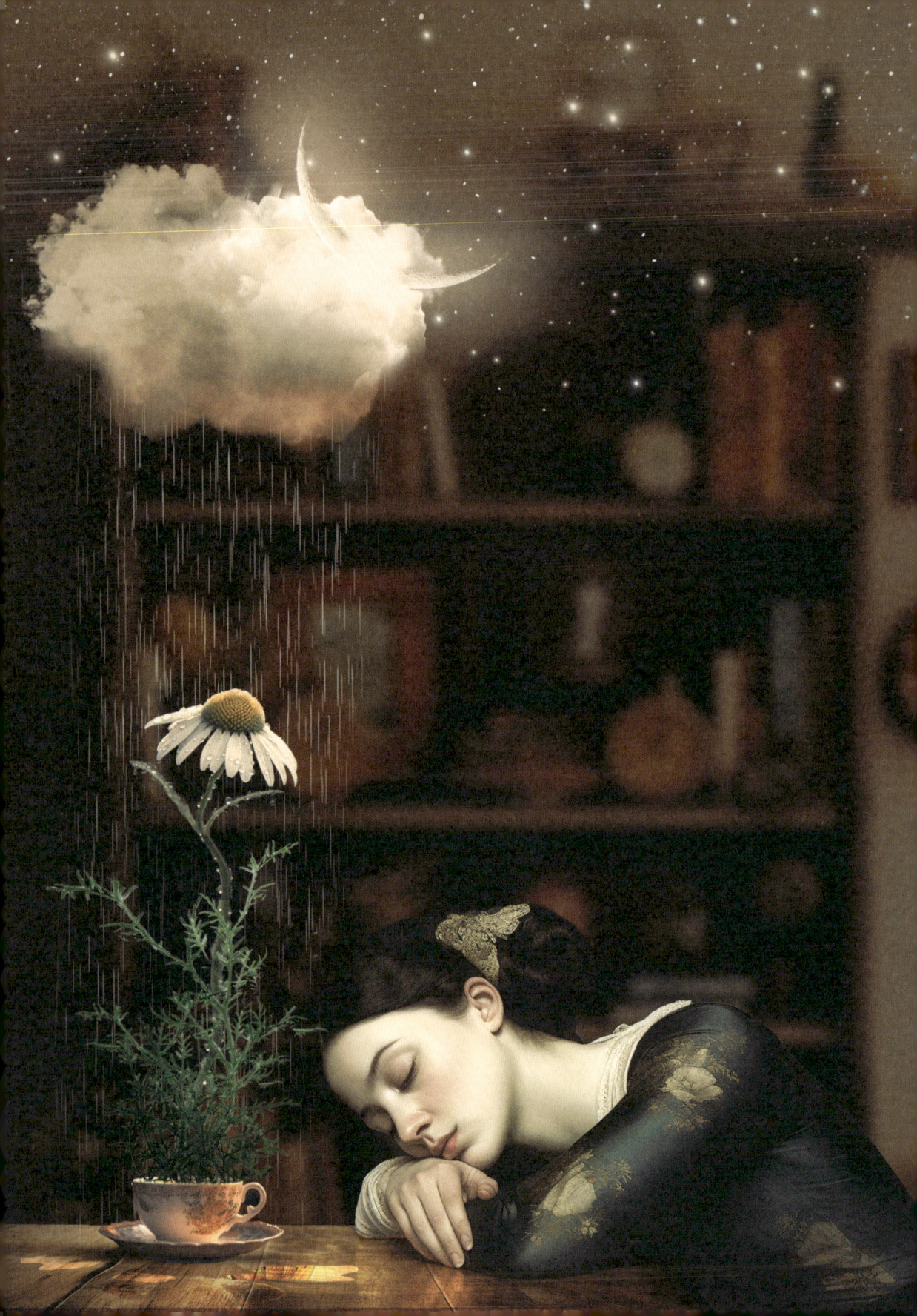

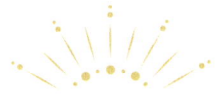

CHAMOMILE

— Matricaria recutita —

Chamomile brings together the wild and the domestic spirits. It grows carried by the wind, a constant nomad. But it is also a symbol of domestic tranquility, thanks to its unmistakable herbal tea. Its dual nature releases a message that is both strong and gentle: keep your heart light. It is linked to calmness. In phytotherapy, it is known for its relaxing properties and is often used to promote sleep and relieve stress. Its active ingredients, such as apigenin, work to calm the nervous system, promoting a sense of inner calm. It has anti-inflammatory and antispasmodic properties. It is also used to relieve gastrointestinal disorders and as a natural remedy for skin irritations or sunburn. Its flowers are small, with white and yellow petals arranged radially around a convex center, and the leaves are slender, threadlike, and bright green. From a magical point of view, it promotes serenity of mind.

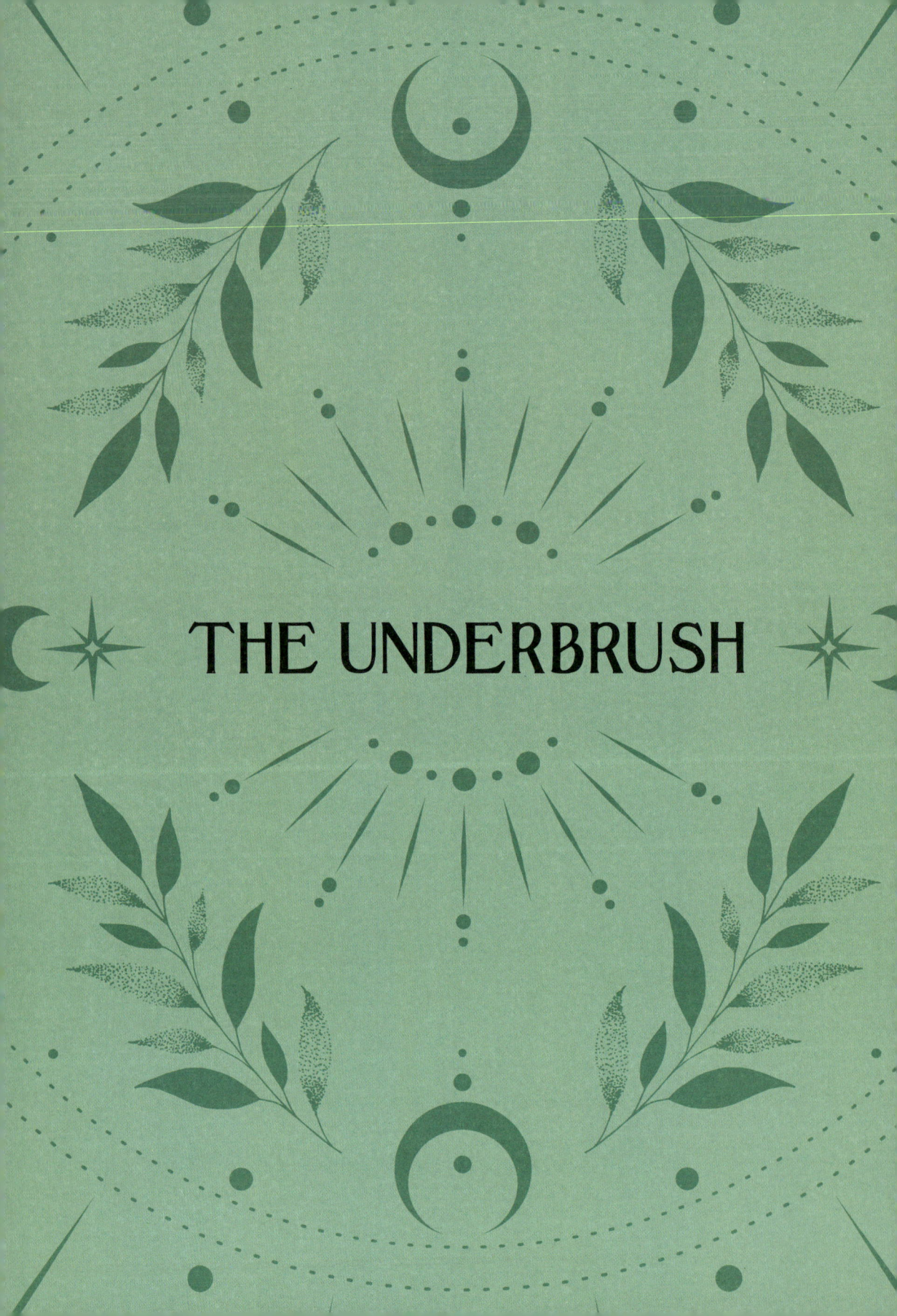

THE UNDERBRUSH

There is a place in the heart of the woods where the green soul of the forest pulses: the underbrush. It is a hidden world, where sunlight penetrates the path in a different way. Entering the underbrush gives the same feeling as entering the doorway of an ancient cathedral. The underbrush possesses a sacred dimension. It is one of those places where whispering comes naturally. The temperature changes, it becomes cooler, and it smells of wet earth, moss, and fir, which tastes like lemon. Here you can find secret passages or magical creatures, such as fairies, who sometimes leave a magical imprint to follow when they pass by. The same is true of a circle of mushrooms, which, when arranged in a precise and mysterious order, is said to be a sign of the fairy's dance, a magical dance that stops time for those who participate. If you happen to join the fairy dance, you return to reality months or years later, like the characters of many fairy tales. The underbrush is a threshold, and, because of that, it is a magical place, where anything seems possible: finding hidden treasure, talking to a fox, or picking up a fairy's glove. It is the forest witch's favorite place, her sanctuary, where she works and gathers herbs and plants with mysterious protective and healing powers. It is here that she meets her animal guides: the owl, wolf, and hare, the sole guardians of her secrets.

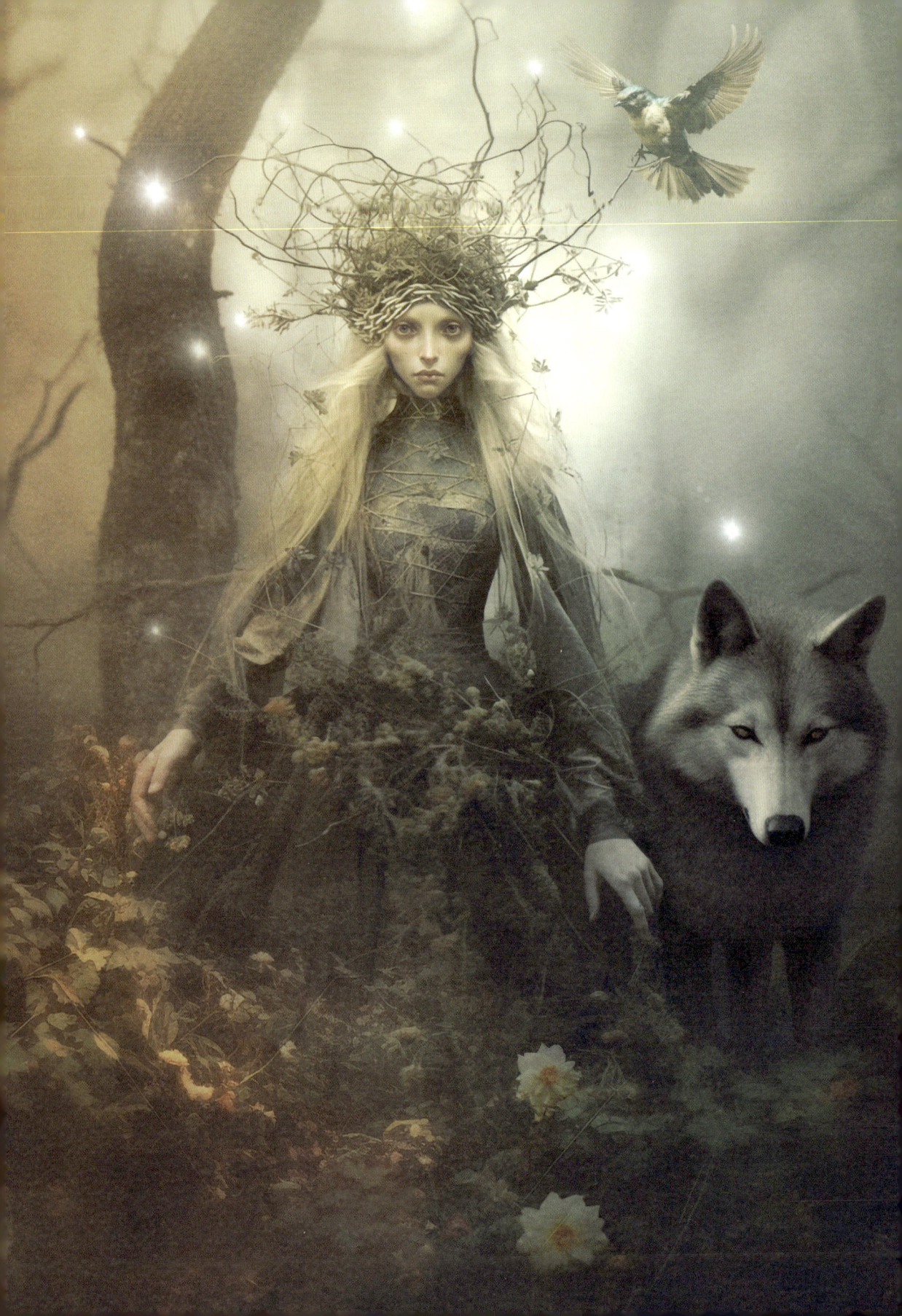

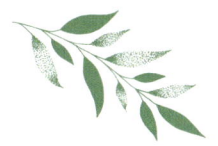
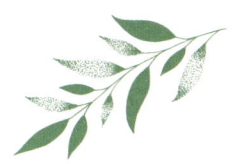

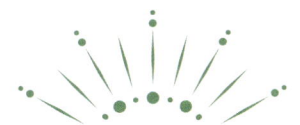

THE FOREST WITCH

—

The forest witch knows the underbrush like the back of her hand, a magical map, which always takes her where she needs to be. She is a solitary witch, but she operates in close contact with the forest and its inhabitants, the animals and fairies.

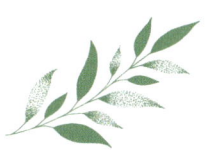
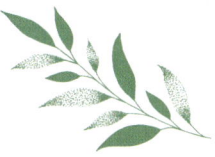

he gnomes and fairies know her well, and she knows them. They inhabit the same worlds, visible and invisible, and take care of them. More than any other witch, she embodies the wild and untamed nature of the forest. She knows when is the right time to harvest comfrey root and when to leave fertilizer and rose hip and hawthorn honey, silent guardians of the two worlds.

Her specialty is the creation of amulets and talismans, which come from the wisdom of nature. She immerses herself in the energy of the forest, gathers what she needs, and creates protective talismans against negative energy by weaving strands of herbs. Or she makes amulets to attract prosperity and abundance by placing a shiny stone on the knot of a root.

With the secret treasures of the forest, inspired by those of shamans, she makes her medicine bags, pouches that embody the magic and essence of the forest. These precious pouches are made from handwoven strands of plant fibers, following the witch's ancient art of weaving. Inside the medicine bag of the forest, the forest witch keeps her personal trove of magical and sacred objects, carefully collected during her searches in the underbrush. There are aromatic roots with a gentle fragrance, herbs with healing properties, stones gathered along secret paths, leaves that look like fine fabrics, feathers of singing birds, and many other small treasures, such as river pebbles or crystals, which are connected to the realms of air and water. Each object has symbolic meaning and magical power: herbs for potions and incense, stones for magical amulets, feathers for flying between worlds, and bones and pebbles for returning to one's roots and not losing one's way home.

> The forest witch uses the forest medicine bag—a powerful tool that can channel the dialogue between the wild and the everyday—during her magical practices, and she uses the objects it contains with respect and care. And there, after fulfilling her enchantment, the forest witch returns home.

Behind her, the leaves of the oak tree have just fallen, delicate on the dark earth, and farther away a wolf watches her as it distances itself. It is her magical and faithful companion, which can live at a distance while still being close when she needs it.

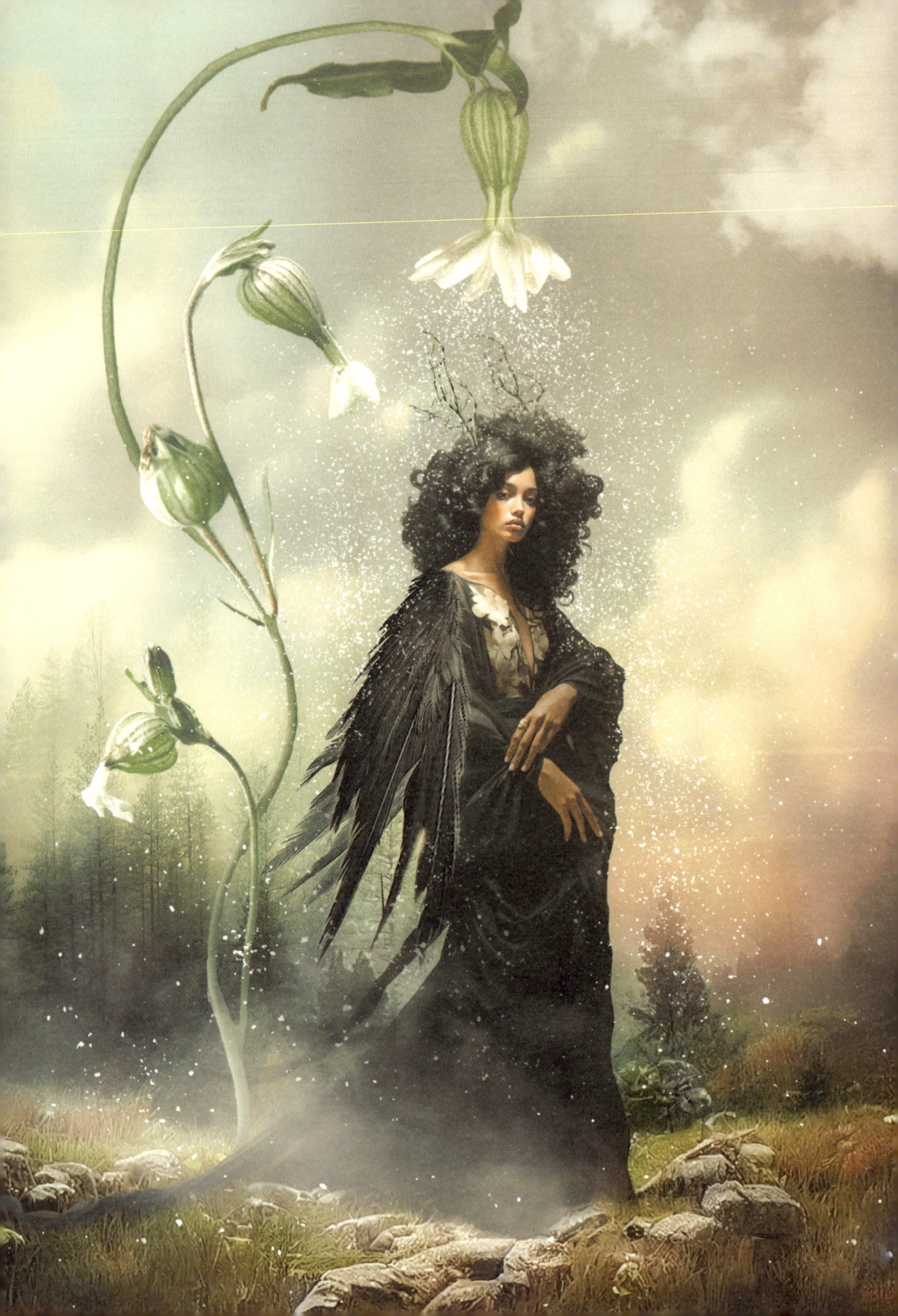

CATCHFLY

– Silene vulgaris
or Silene alba –

Catchfly, also called campion, grows near the woods and can be easily recognized by its leaves, which are opposing, oval, and lanceolate, and its small flowers, which are white and bulbous. Vitamin C, saponins, and mucilage are its most important nutritional values, which therefore should be eaten raw or steamed for a few minutes. Its tasty flavor is reminiscent of freshly picked green peas. But catchfly is also known for its emollient and soothing properties. In folk tradition, it has always been used for its digestive properties. Infusions prepared from its leaves and flowers can aid digestion and soothe gastrointestinal disorders. Discovering where a catchfly plant grows is a gift, as you can find it in the same spot the next year. The plant's name comes from Silenus, companion of Bacchus, who is said to have had a bulging belly just like the little flower. It is connected to clairvoyance, intuition, and a wild spirit.

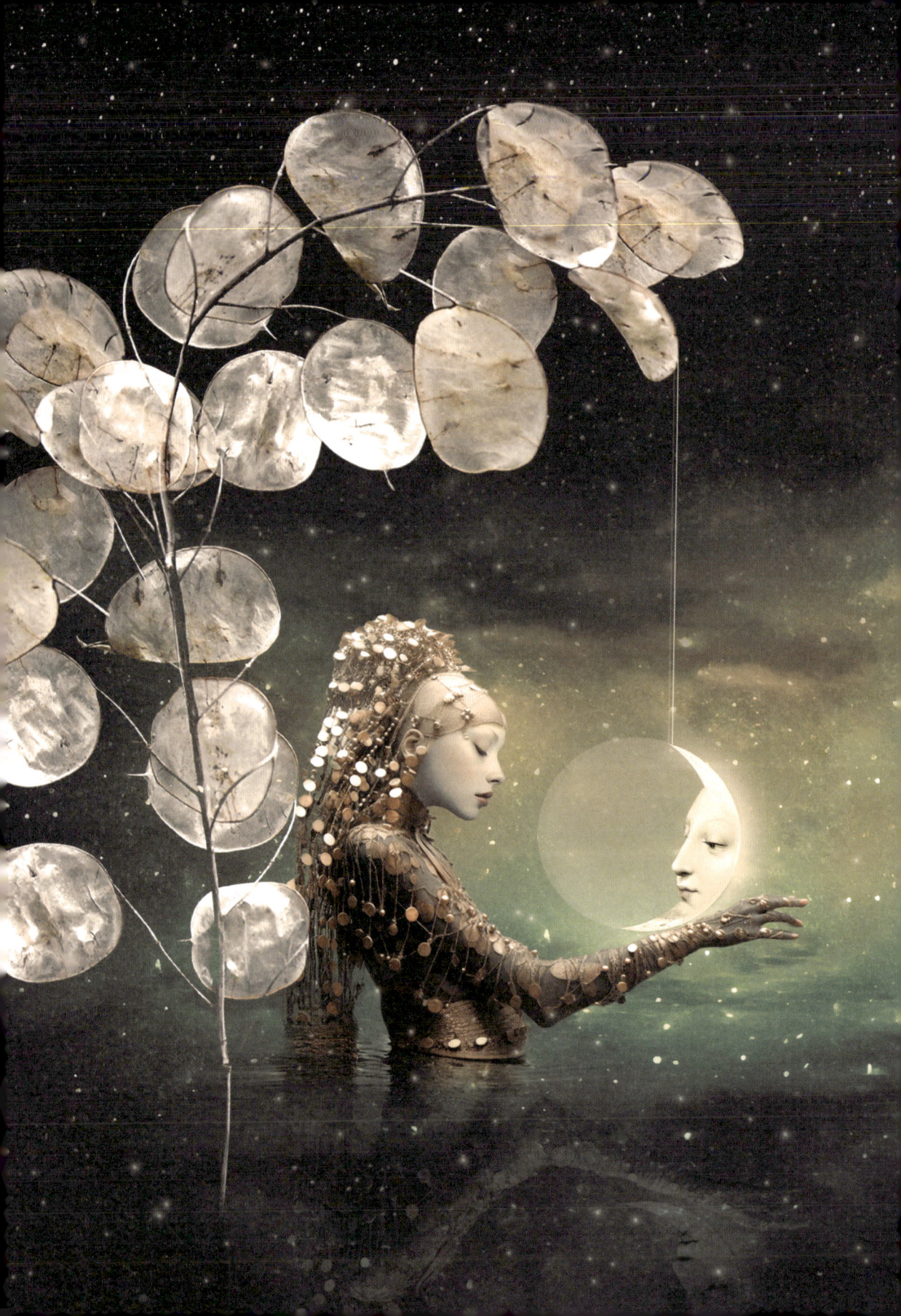

HONESTY

— LUNARIA ANNUA —

There is a plant in the underbrush that, when it bears fruit in late summer, is filled with small, silver moons. This is honesty, whose iridescent medallions hold its seeds. You recognize it by its bright pink flowers, among the first to appear in spring. It is also known as "Pope's money" because of the coin shape of its fruit. It has heart-shaped leaves with serrated edges. The florets are edible and can be eaten like broccoli; when blanched and sautéed with garlic and chili peppers, they make a unique side dish with a sharp, bitter flavor. The fruits, when still green, have a delicious spicy flavor and can be added raw on salads or pickled. The flowers can also be used to decorate spring dishes, cold pastas, and risottos. Its connection with the moon is evident, especially when the fruit dries and releases its seeds, revealing a transparent membrane like a moonbeam.

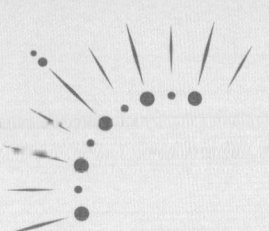

– MAGICAL USES –

Honesty is associated with prosperity and abundance in many folk traditions. Its silvery pods are considered a symbol of wealth and good fortune, and in magical practices they are used as amulets or talismans to invoke abundance in people's lives. It is said that keeping an honesty pod in your home or carrying one with you can promote wealth and prosperity. Due to its round shape linking it to the moon, it was offered to lunar deities for protection against evil spirits and poverty. Also connected to honesty and the ability to be consistent with who you are, it shines its own light because it knows its soul deeply, knows what it wants, and teaches you to always find your way home.

Full Moon Incense

YOU WILL NEED:

- ✻ *Honesty fruits (dried)*
- ✻ *Myrrh resin*
- ✻ *Dried lavender*
- ✻ *Mortar and pestle*

You can prepare this incense on the night of a full moon. Find a quiet, serene place where you can fully focus on the incense, and begin by drawing a magic circle around you to create a sacred, protected space. Take the honesty fruits and gently grind them in the mortar, focusing your intention during the process. Visualize the moonlight reflecting in the fruits, turning them into a magical powder. Add the myrrh resin to the mortar and continue grinding carefully, combining the purifying and protective energy of the myrrh with the power of the honesty. Add the dried lavender to the mortar and grind it to a smooth, fragrant mixture. Transfer the mixture to a glass container and store it in a cool, dark place until you're ready to use it.

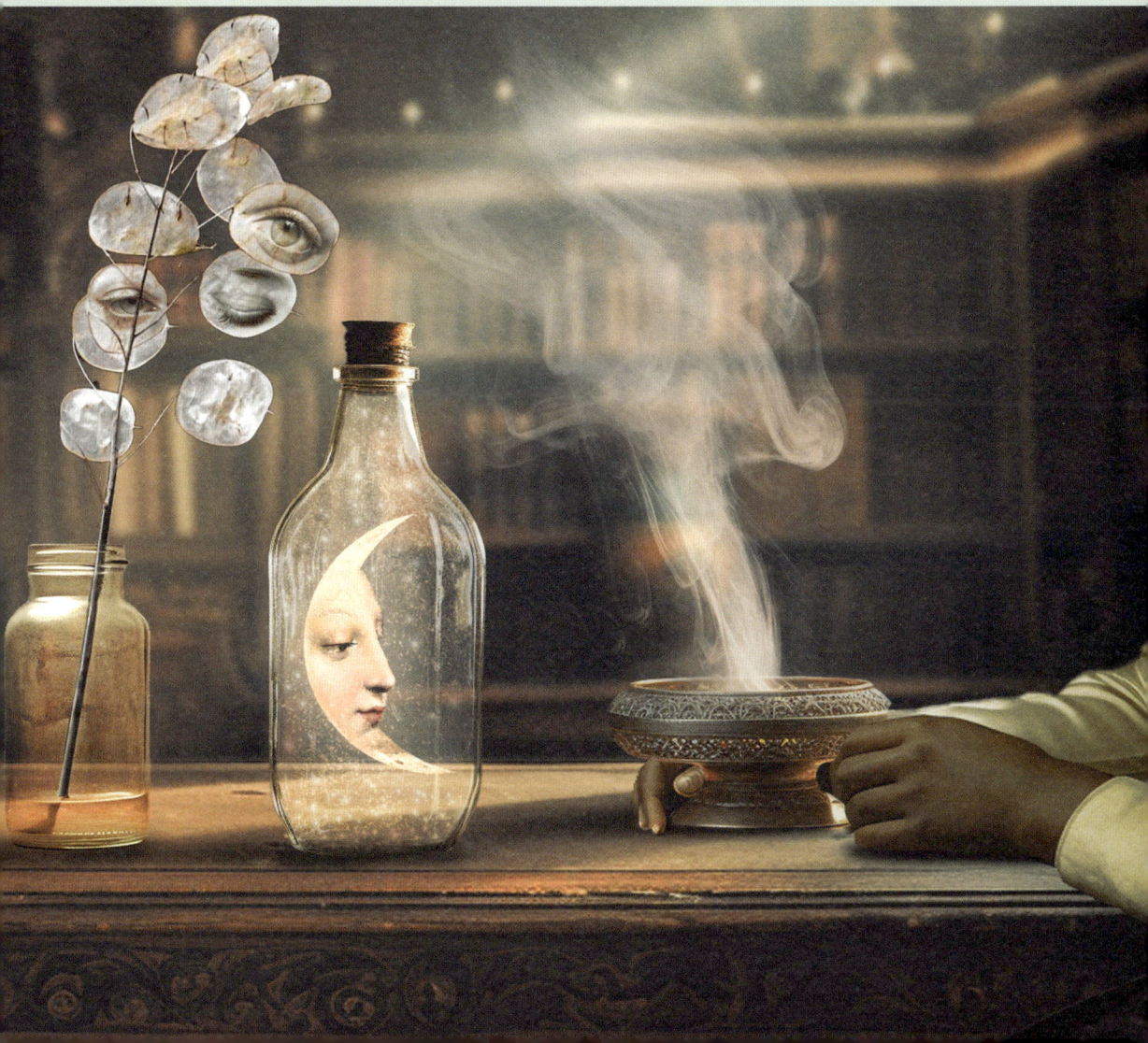

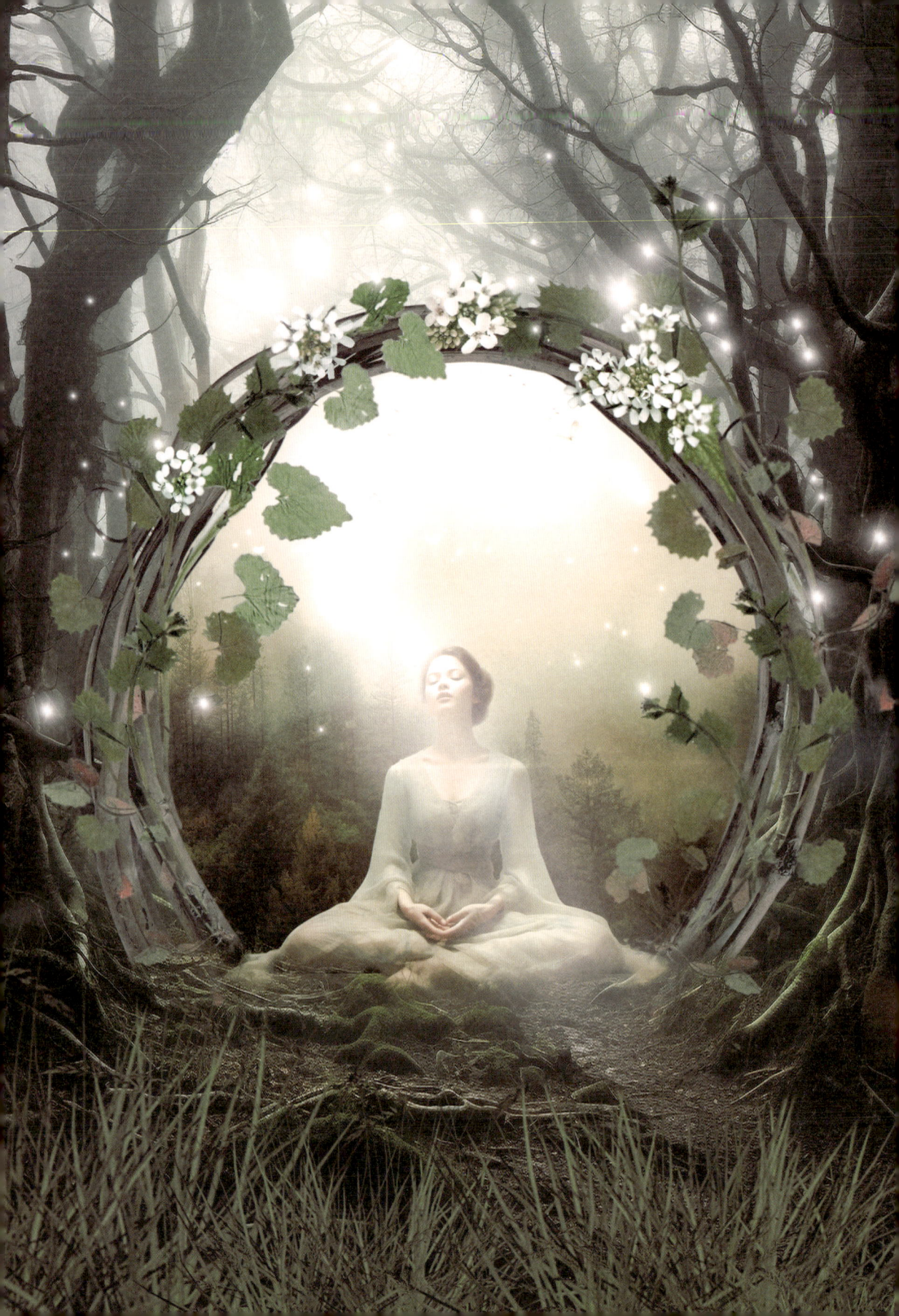

GARLIC MUSTARD

— ALLIARIA PETIOLATA —

Garlic mustard is a sister to honesty and has white flowers and a distinct garlic aroma. It grows in the underbrush in shady, moist places. It can be recognized not only by its smell but also by its heart-shaped leaves with serrated edges. The plant, valued for its unique flavor and nutritious properties, is suitable for those who do not digest garlic but love its flavor. Its nickname is "Jack-by-the-hedge." Plants that live on the edge and mark boundaries are very important from a magical point of view. As guardians of the threshold, they protect and ward off negativity. The plant is also called devil-by-the-hedge, which refers to a story told to children to make them return home: when the *Alliaria* leaves begin to give off their strong smell at dusk, it is time to return home because the devil is coming. Because of its pungent scent, garlic mustard is associated with fire and Beltane rites. You can weave a wreath of flowers to celebrate the arrival of summer.

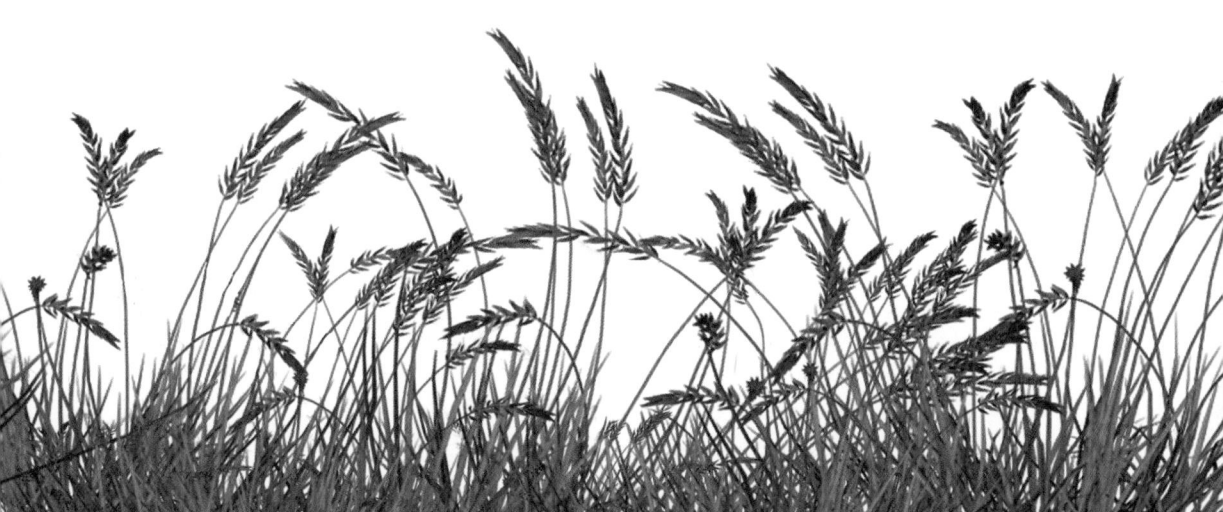

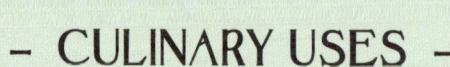

– CULINARY USES –

Garlic mustard holds many beneficial nutritional properties. Rich in vitamin C, vitamin A, calcium, and iron, this wild plant can contribute to a balanced diet by providing important nutrients. Its leaves, with their characteristic aroma of fresh garlic, can be used in a variety of ways: raw in salads for a slightly spicy taste and a hint of fresh garlic; finely chopped and added to sauces, soups, or vegetable dishes; or in a tasty pesto to spread on bread or in pasta.

Pasta with Garlic Mustard Pesto

YOU WILL NEED:

- *2 cups of fresh garlic mustard leaves*
- *1/2 cup of fresh basil leaves*
- *A handful of walnuts or pine nuts*
- *1/4 cup of grated cheese (parmesan or pecorino)*
or nutritional yeast for vegans
- *2 garlic cloves*
- *Juice of 1/2 lemon*
- *1/2 cup of extra virgin olive oil*
- *Salt and pepper to taste*
- *10 ounces (300 g) of pasta (best if spaghetti or penne)*

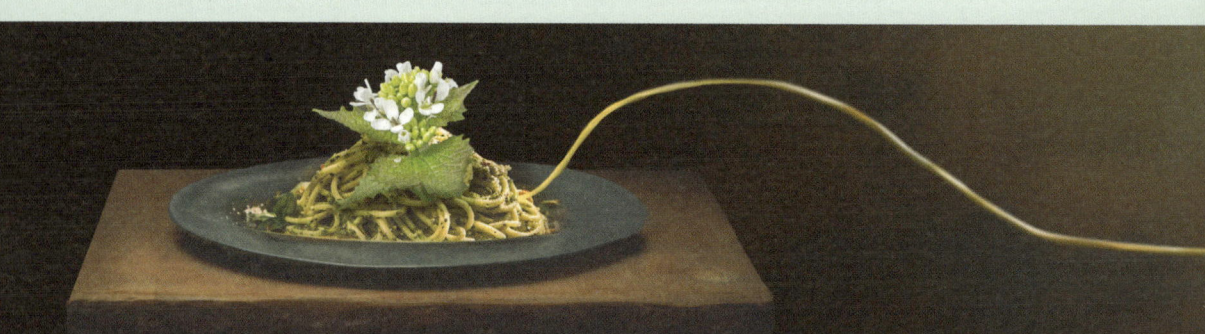

In a pot of salted water, boil the pasta. Meanwhile, thoroughly rinse the garlic mustard and basil leaves. In a blender or food processor, add the leaves, walnuts or pine nuts, grated cheese or nutritional yeast, garlic, and lemon juice. Blend until smooth. Gradually add the extra virgin olive oil while the blender is running, until a creamy sauce is obtained. Adjust salt and pepper to suit your taste. Drain the pasta—*al dente* is recommended—and toss with the garlic mustard pesto. Serve the pasta with a sprinkling of grated cheese or nutritional yeast and fresh garlic mustard leaves.

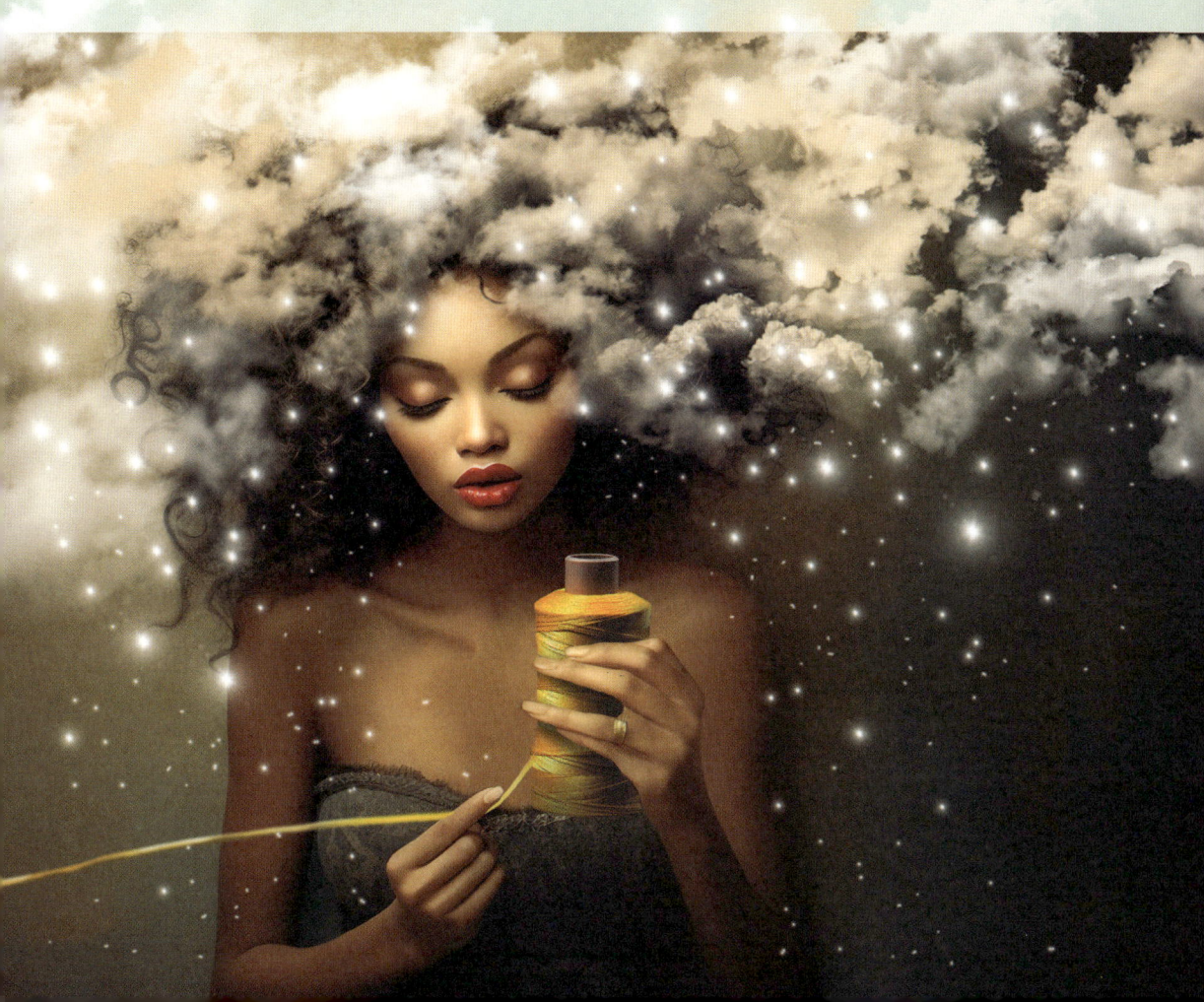

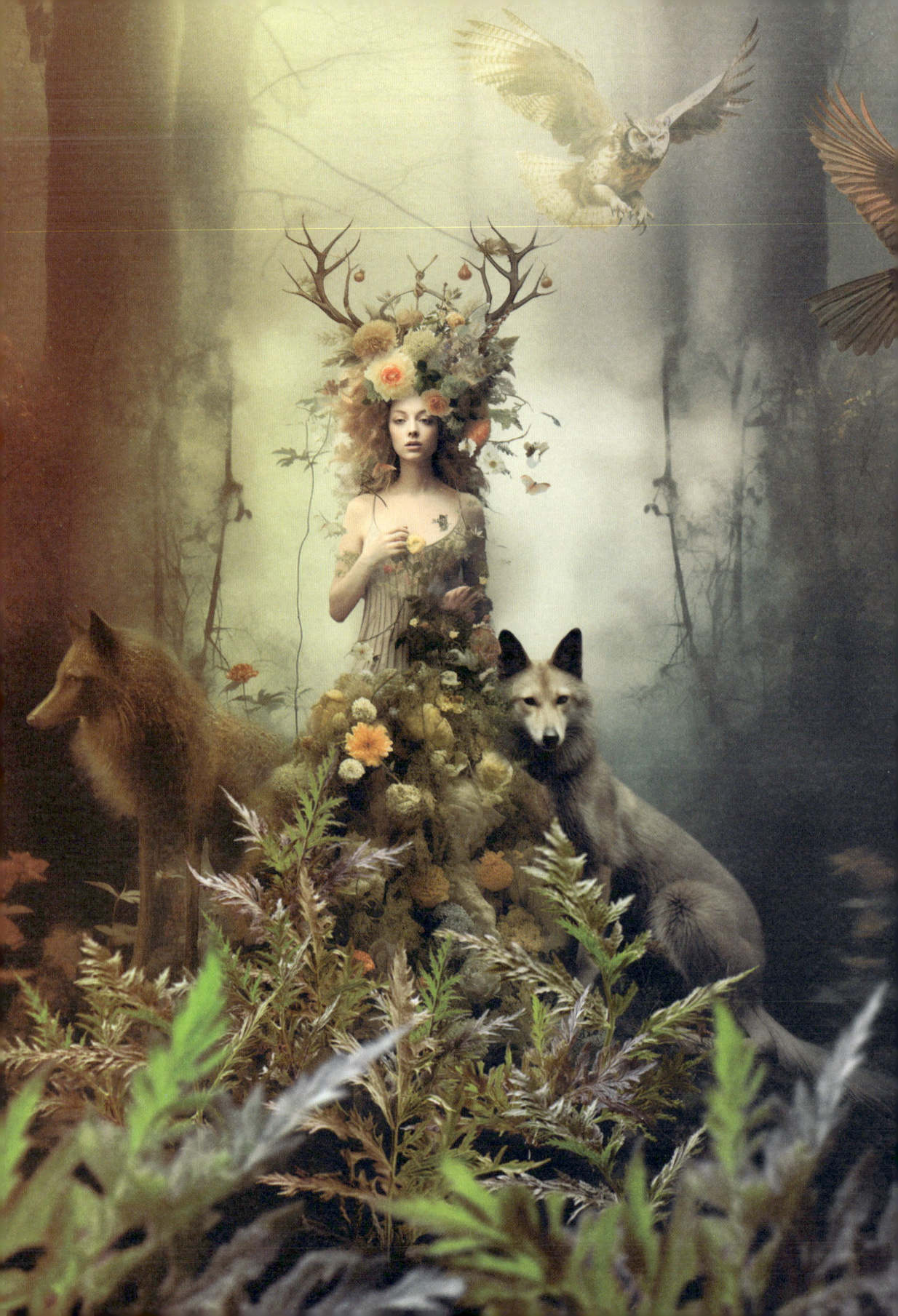

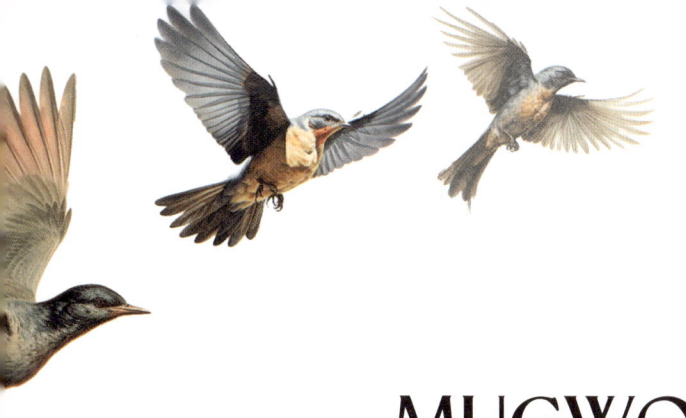

MUGWORT

– Artemisia vulgaris –

Mugwort, with its silvery leaves shining in the moonlight, populates the underbrush. It is dedicated to the moon and to Artemis, hence the name, the patron goddess of the woods, of bears, and of the untamed spirit. Its aromatic scent is unmistakable, and it accompanies you whenever you go into the woods. In phytotherapy, some species are used for their aromatic and medicinal properties, which can promote digestion, relieve menstrual disorders, and support the immune system. However, it is important to consult a doctor before using it, as it contains a mildly toxic substance called thujone. According to folk tradition, mugwort is linked to the dreamworld. Keeping a few leaves under your pillow would foster prophetic dreams. When burned as incense, on the other hand, it can induce a state of relaxation and open-mindedness, sparking deep visions.

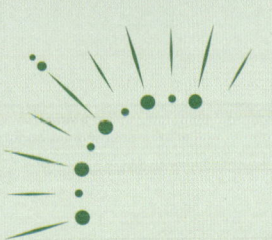

– COSMETIC USES –

Artemisia, with its energetic and therapeutic properties, is a plant that can be particularly beneficial for the female womb and cycle. Its calming and invigorating properties can help relieve discomfort and promote a harmonious balance. Its subtle energy is in touch with the moon and the deep spirit of sisterhood, in connection with the energy of the goddess Artemis. A macerated oil can be created with its leaves, which is excellent for massaging the belly.

Moon Oil

YOU WILL NEED:

- ✿ *1 cup of carrier oil (almond or jojoba oil)*
- ✿ *2 spoonfuls of dried mugwort leaves*
- ✿ *5 drops of lavender essential oil*
- ✿ *3 drops of clary sage essential oil*
- ✿ *3 drops of rose essential oil*

Start by pouring the carrier oil into a dark glass jar. Add the dried mugwort leaves to the oil and close the jar tightly. Place the jar in a cool, dark place and let the macerated mugwort oil sit for two to four weeks. Shake the bottle gently every two to three days to help extract the properties of the mugwort. After the resting time, strain the oil using a fine strainer or paper filter to separate the leaves. Add the lavender, rose, and clary sage oils to the filtered mugwort oil. Mix well to combine the ingredients. Transfer the resulting oil to a dark glass bottle and store in a cool, dark place.

HOW TO USE IT

Apply a small amount of oil to the palms of your hands, and warm the oil by rubbing your hands together. Massage the abdomen clockwise in gentle circular motions, focusing on the lower abdomen and the area around the navel. During the massage, breathe deeply and relax, focusing on the positive sensations you feel and visualizing the balance of your belly. You can repeat the massage once or twice a day, depending on your needs and the symptoms you wish to relieve.

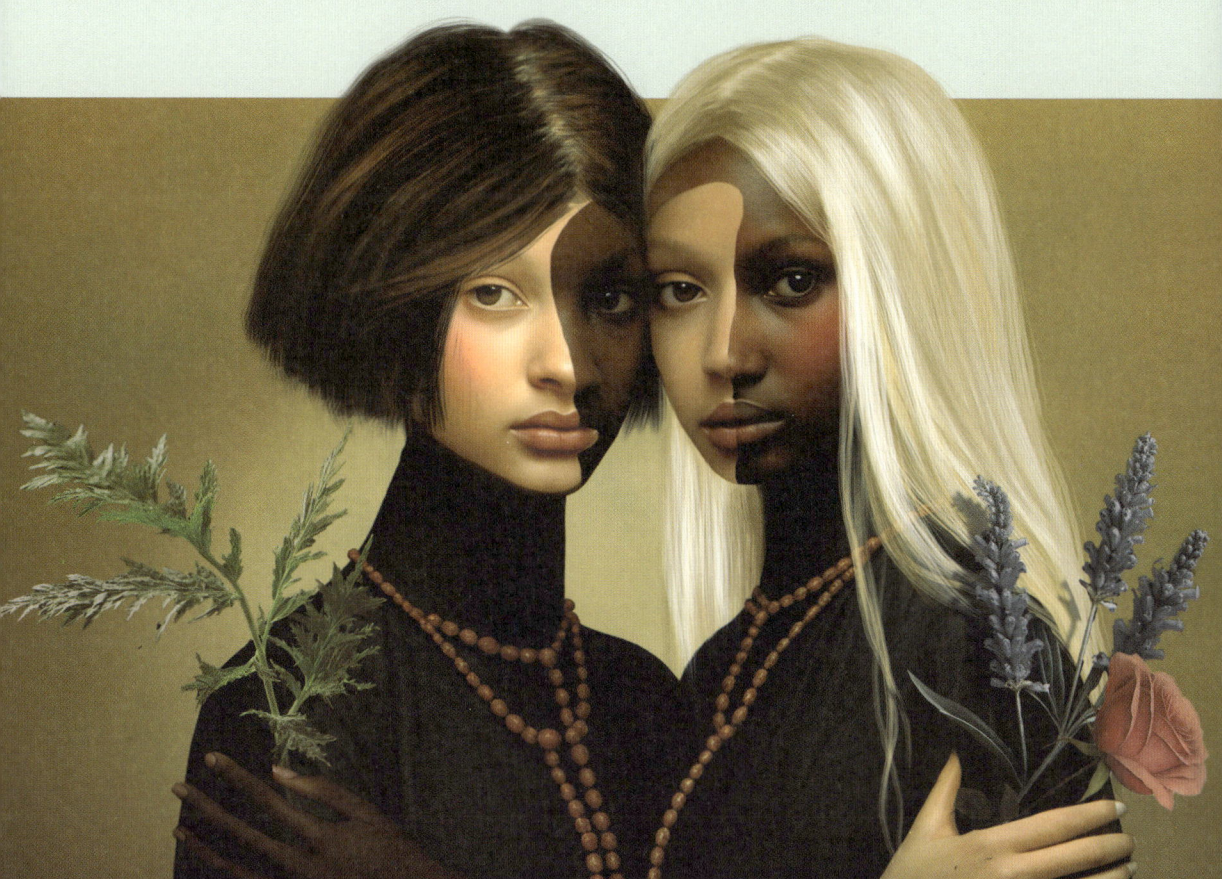

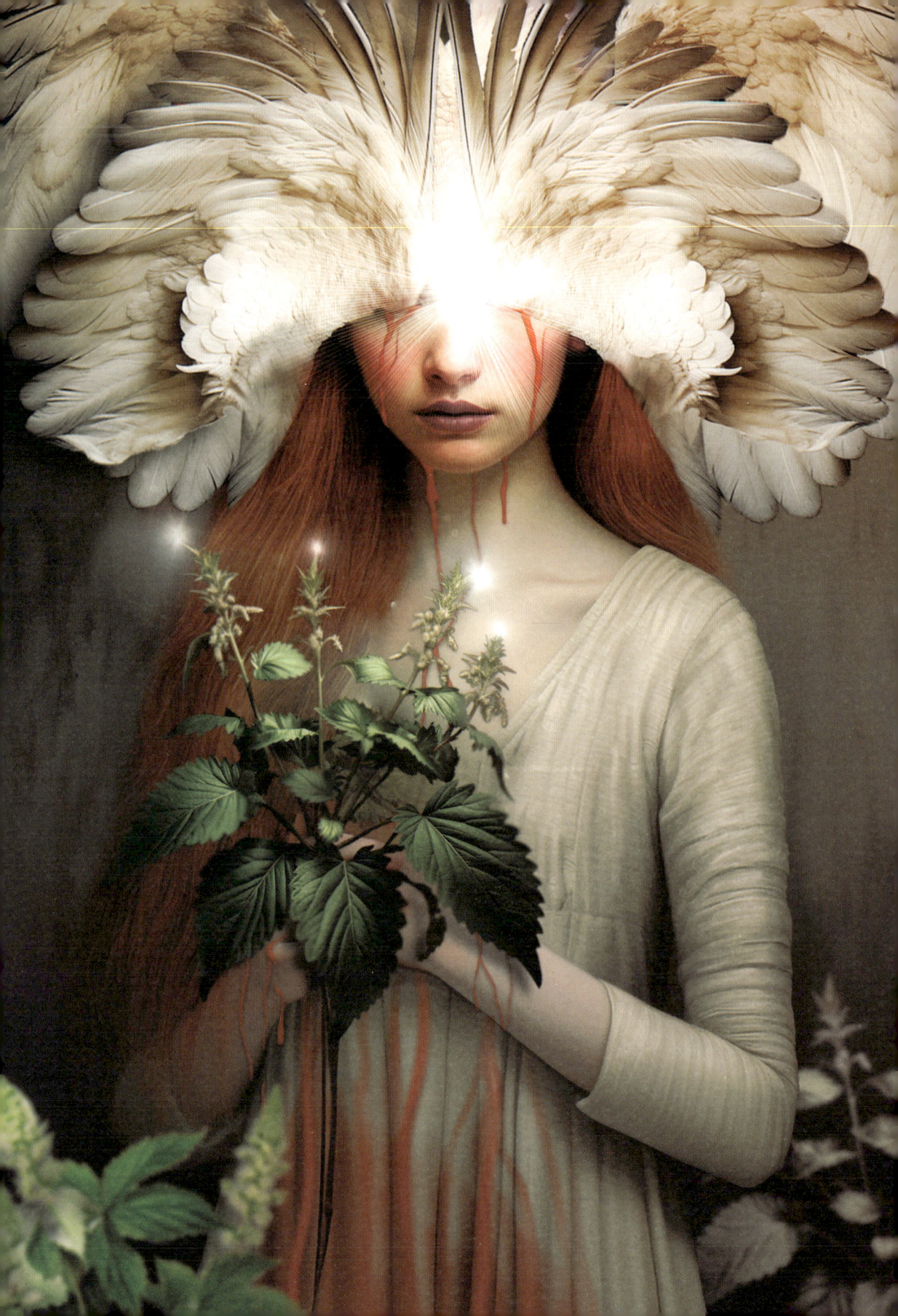

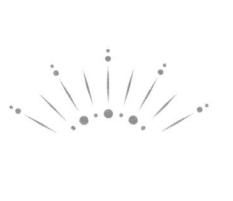

NETTLE

— Urtica dioica —

Even in its humility, nettle is one of the most powerful wild plants. It grows at the edge of the forest and, as long as you don't brush against it, it can go unnoticed. If touched, however, it reveals its nature and releases its famous irritant: nettle stings, marking its space and reminding you that everyone is unique, even if it doesn't show on the surface. A useful plant for metabolizing iron, as it acts on ferritin metabolism, it is good for the blood, which it regenerates and purifies. In addition, nettle has hematopoietic properties, whereby it can promote the production of red blood cells in the bone marrow, thus helping to increase their number and improve circulation. Its connection with blood puts it in contact with Mars, and, from a magical point of view, it can be used in rituals related to protection, strength, and vitality. It can be used to create protective amulets or as an ingredient in potions or incense to stimulate passion and vital energy.

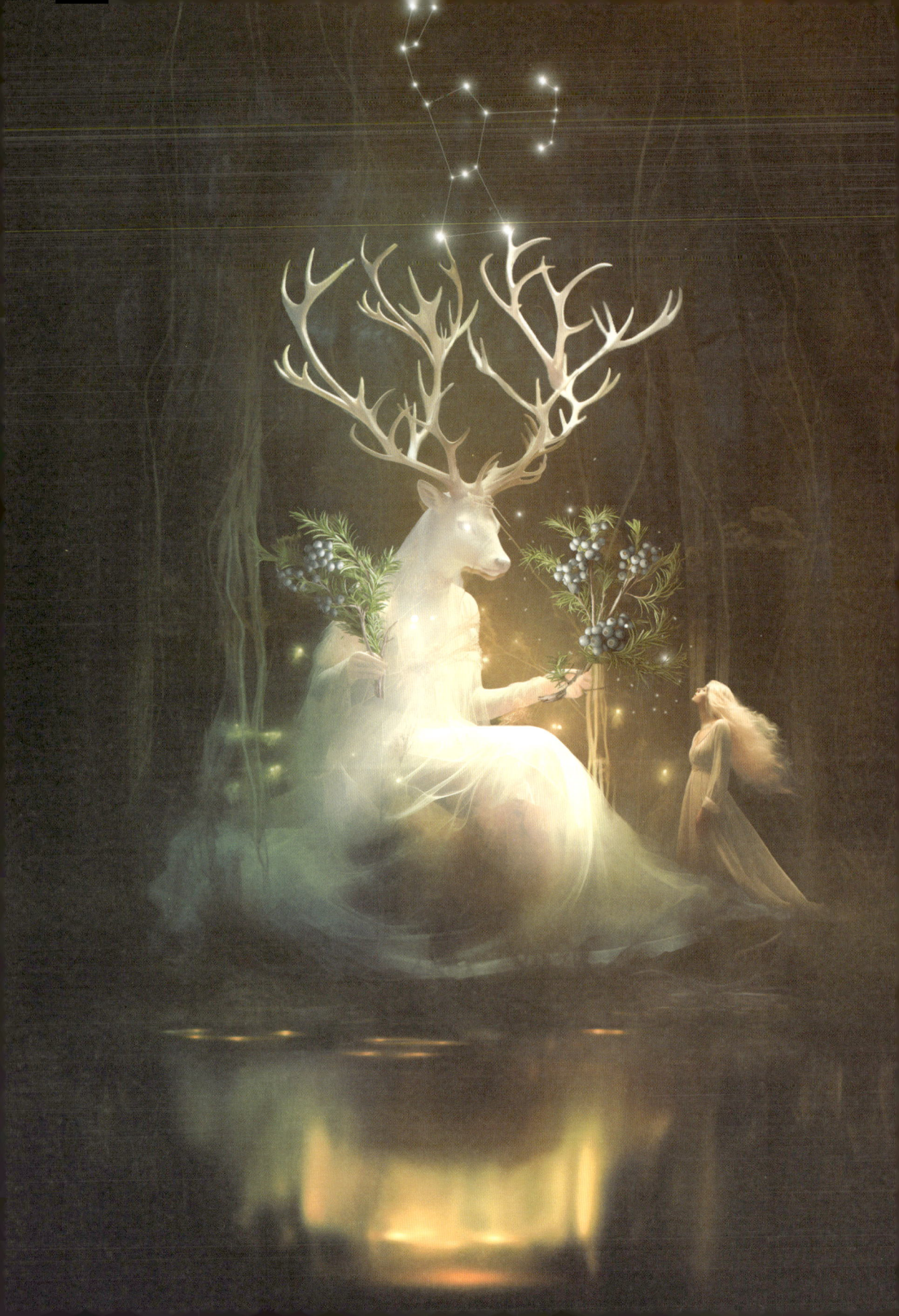

JUNIPER

— JUNIPERUS COMMUNIS —

Juniper is a guardian of the underbrush, a threshold plant between this world and the beyond. It protects the Fair Folk, fairies, and elves. It has needle-shaped leaves and berries ranging from green to deep blue, as unripe and ripe berries can be found together. Many folk traditions attribute protective abilities to it. Throwing its needles on the floor or hanging its branches over doors and windows is said to protect a house from evil spirits. When burned, its wood gives off a pleasant aroma and purifies the air. The berries, used as a spice, add a distinctive flavor to many dishes, particularly meats and stews. In herbal medicine, it is known for its diuretic, digestive, and anti-inflammatory properties. The berries are often used in the preparation of decoctions, herbal teas, or infusions that can aid digestion and diuresis, and can relieve gastrointestinal disorders. Warning: do not use during pregnancy or breastfeeding, or if you have kidney problems.

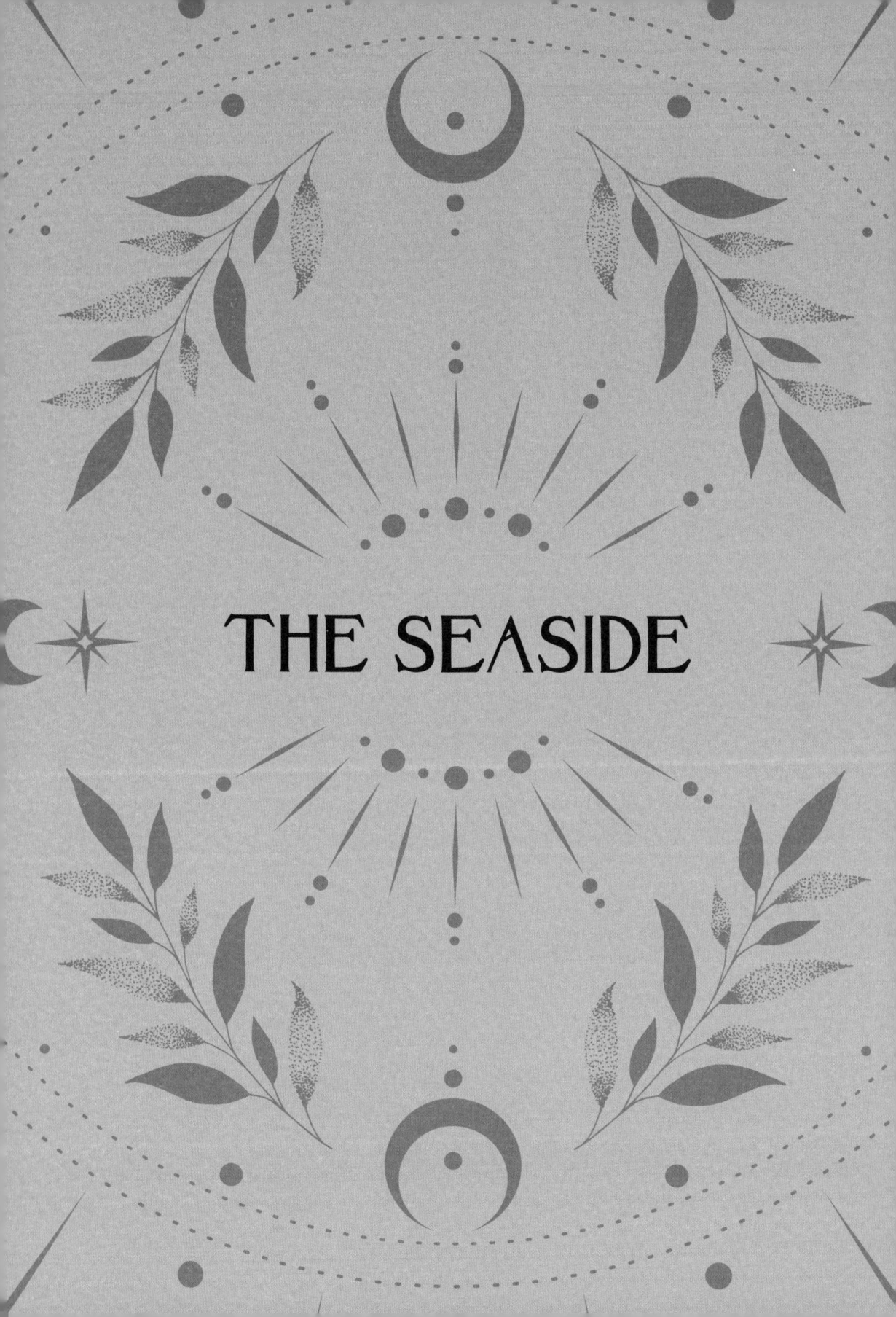

THE SEASIDE

The seaside is a special place that retains its charm at all times of the year, even if it is experienced by most in the summer. Walking along the seaside—with your eyes full of light and your gaze wandering to the bright horizon—is magic in itself. You can soak in the beauty and feel it resonate, with every step you take, as an invitation to discover the mysteries, hidden treasures in the waves. The seaside is a full sensory experience; the fine sand, scorching and dry or wet and cool; the salty scent of shells found among the waves; the caress of a soft seagull feather found on the beach and the helichrysum bushes, to be rubbed gently with your fingers to release the unmistakable smell of licorice and summer. The plants that grow near the sea are intoxicating, and they immediately take you back to the summers of your childhood. The memory is part of the waterfront, as is the joy of being able to experience such spontaneous and simple contact with the grandeur of nature. It is a place of openness and infinite possibilities, and it is here that our hearts open to infinity, before the greatness of the sea. Since time immemorial, the sea has held mysteries: old pirate galleons sunk centuries ago, magical plants that grow only underwater, and mermaids with iridescent tails spotted here and there by astonished observers. Often, witches live near the sea, in wooden houses overlooking the beach, on the door of which dream catchers woven with shells tinkle lightly, inviting you to enter.

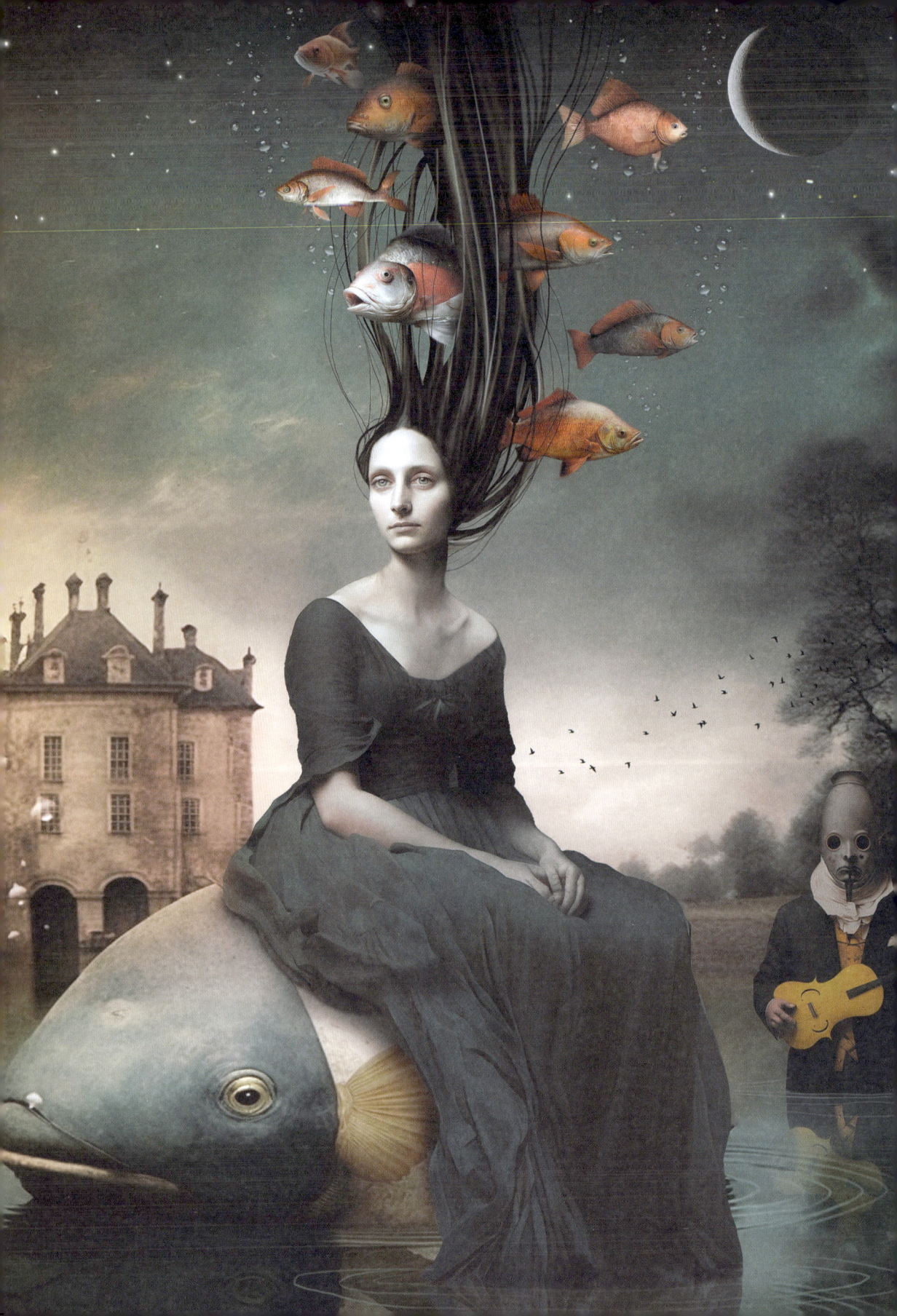

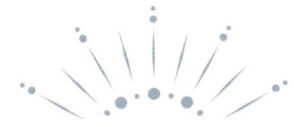

THE SIREN
WITCH

—

There she is, waiting for you in
her wooden house, looking out to
sea. Her hair, long and flowing like
brown seaweed, resembles waves,
and her house smells of wild fennel
and rosemary. On the doorstep,
numerous succulent plants welcome
those who pass by for advice or to
contemplate the sunset.

he siren witch protects the sea and its creatures. She knows that everything is one and that the marine environment is a delicate ecosystem that must be taken care of. She is deeply connected to the primordial power of water, which nourishes her with a unique magical energy.

She is symbiotic with the sea and its depths, and through her connection with water the mermaid witch is able to explore the secrets of this element, sense its energy flows, and channel them for her purposes.

She intuits the power of the waves, the mysterious energy of sea whirlpools, and the deep calm of serene waters. She knows that water is the symbol of life and regeneration, capable of creating and destroying, healing and purifying.

Using sea plants, she can heal people, both from wounds of the soul and wounds of the heart. At the same time, she can evoke the power of sea storms, moving the waves to protect the coasts or repel those who threaten the balance of the oceans.

Perhaps, in the past, she was a mermaid. Her voice is peculiar, magical, as she has the power to modulate the waves of the sea, and to communicate with the creatures that inhabit it. Her song is an invocation and a prayer, vibrating with natural power and reaching the center of your heart. In her small home, you can find many magical objects: extremely rare and shiny pearls like drops of crystal clear water, which she uses to create pendants that bring good luck and protection; precious jewelry that carries the essence of the sea; and enchanted shells, treasures that tell stories of the sea as if they were keys to other worlds. She collects them and stores them in velvet pouches or carved wooden boxes that carefully guard their most precious secrets. As a solitary witch, she is also very attached to animals, especially those that inhabit the sea. For example, she can communicate with dolphins, who bring her messages from the depths of the ocean and offer her their guidance during her travels between worlds.

But the greatest power of this witch lies in her compassion. Some swear to have seen her emerge from the water at twilight, transform into a siren with an iridescent fish tail, and dive into the deep heart of the sea.

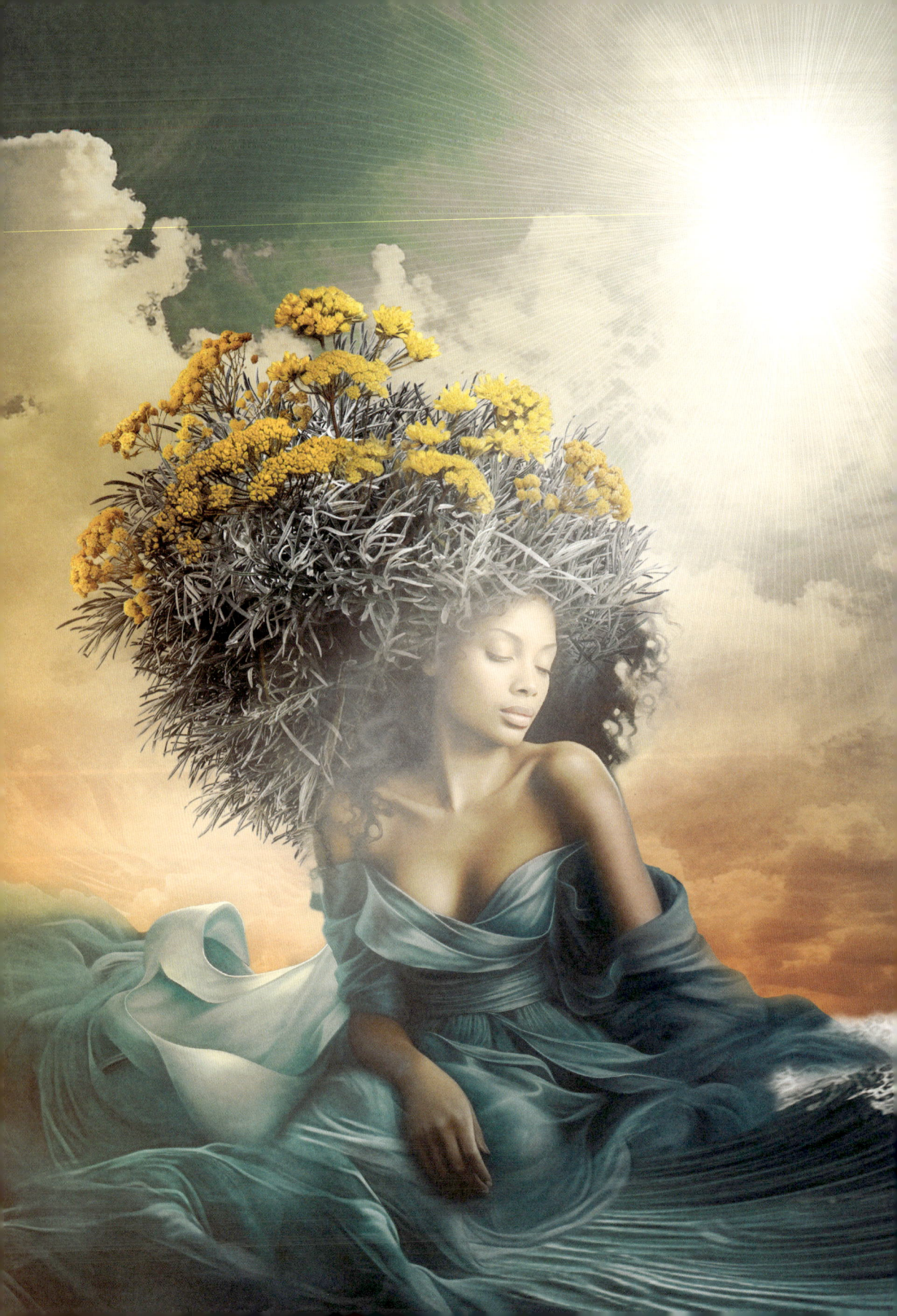

HELICHRYSUM

— HELICHRYSUM ITALICUM —

Helichrysum holds the soul of summer. You can find it near the beach, exposed to the sun, on which it seems to feed. It is recognizable by its silvery leaves and yellow flowers gathered at the apex of the stem, which remain intact even when dried. It has a distinctive licorice scent that immediately evokes the sea and the feeling of sand between your fingers. Its flowers are rich in essential oils with anti-inflammatory, healing, and soothing properties. Its phytotherapeutic uses include effectiveness in treating skin conditions, promoting tissue healing, and reducing inflammation, contributing to skin regeneration. One common name is immortelle because of its tendency to remain intact, hence it is a symbol of fidelity, longevity, and lasting memories. Its scientific name, *Helichrysum*, is derived from the Greek *helios* (sun) and *chrysos* (gold) and refers to its golden splendor and its role as a light bearer.

– COSMETIC USES –

Because of its soothing properties, helichrysum is especially good for sensitive, irritated, or reddish skin. Helichrysum oleolite can be used to soothe skin irritations such as dermatitis, eczema, and sunburn. It contains antioxidants and active compounds that help fight the signs of skin aging, reducing the appearance of wrinkles and improving skin elasticity. It is an excellent remedy for hair as well. You can apply it to the ends to strengthen them, and to make hair shinier. To enjoy these cosmetic properties, you can use helichrysum-based products such as oils, creams, lotions, or serums. Alternatively, you can make helichrysum oleolite!

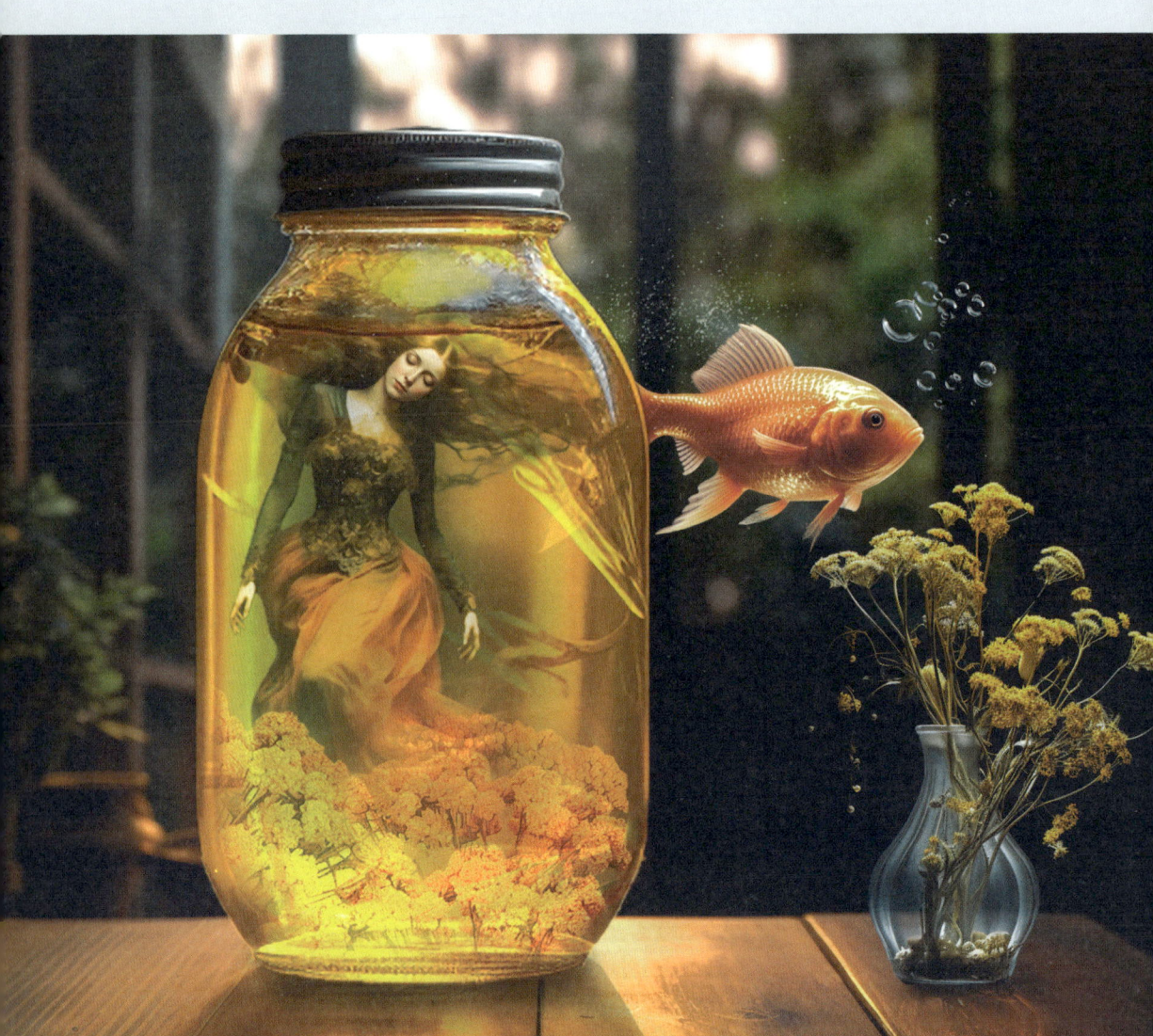

Helichrysum Oleolite

YOU WILL NEED:

- *1 cup of fresh helichrysum flowers and leaves*
- *1 cup of carrier oil (sunflower or olive oil)*

Collect a cup of fresh helichrysum leaves and flowers, making sure to find them in a clean place where no pesticides or chemicals are used. Place the helichrysum leaves and flowers in a clean, dry glass jar. Pour your chosen carrier oil into the jar until the fresh plant is completely covered. Close the jar with gauze secured by a rubber band and shake it gently to mix the oil and plant. Place it in the sunlight, and keep it steeping for four to six weeks. At the end of that time, strain and store in a dark glass bottle. The resulting helichrysum oil can be used as a body oil or massage oil. Apply a small amount of oil to the skin or hair and massage in a gentle motion until fully absorbed.

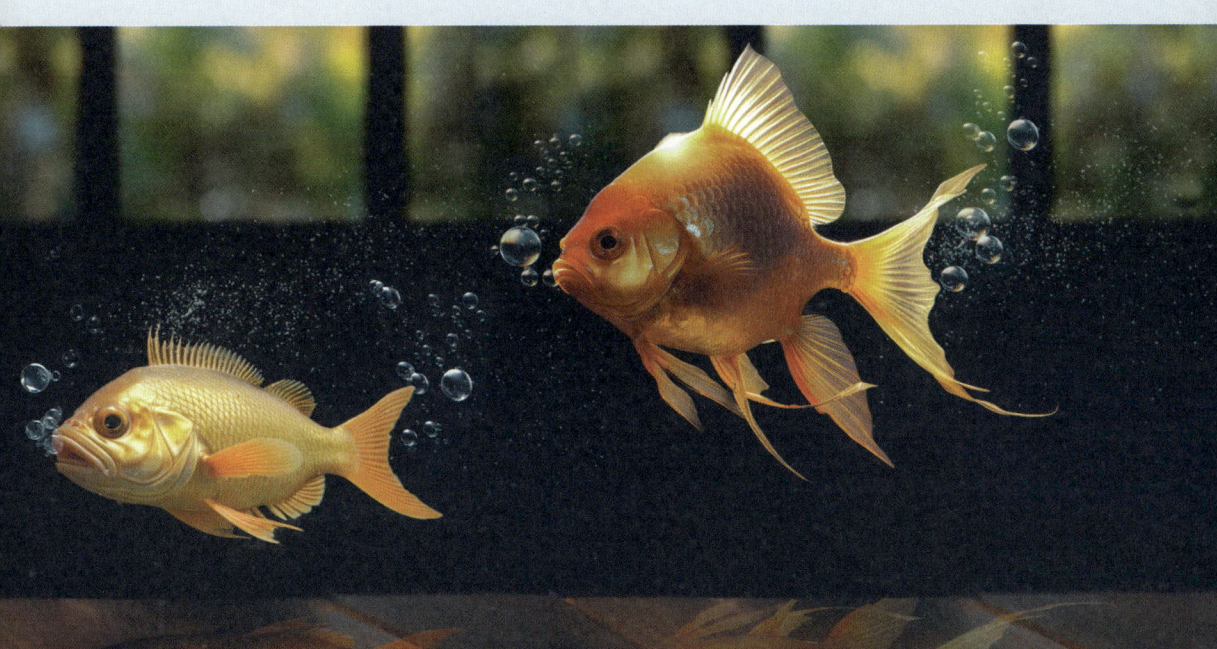

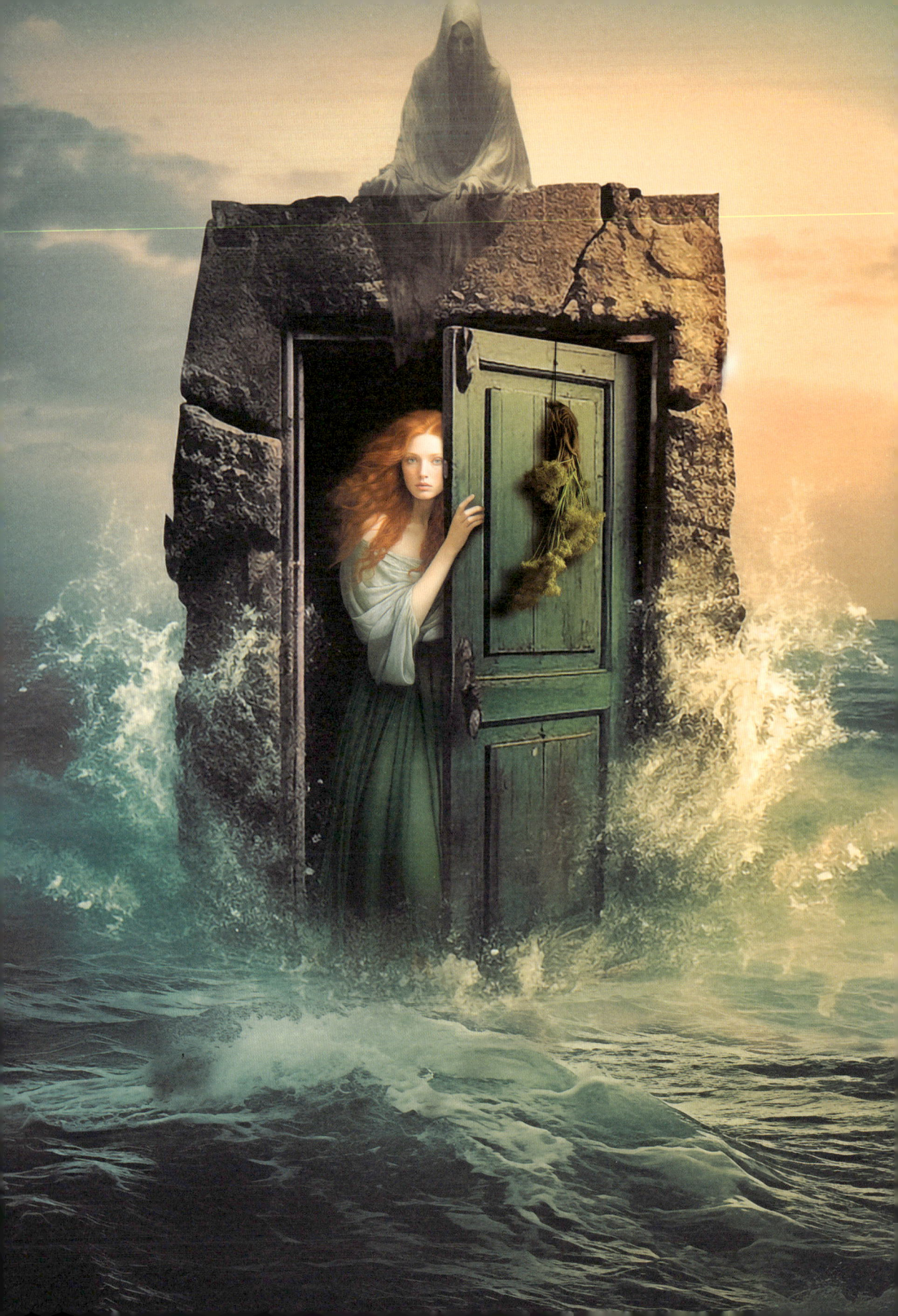

FENNEL

— Foeniculum vulgare var. dulce —

Fennel, or wild fennel, has been used since ancient times as a medicine for many ailments. In fact, fennel and its seeds are widely used in herbal medicine. It grows in sunny, open places and can be recognized by its threadlike fanned leaves and yellow umbrella-shaped flowers. To make sure you don't mistake it, just rub the leaves between your fingers and you will smell its characteristic scent: a mix of anise and wild herbs. Fennel seeds have digestive properties. A fennel seed herbal tea aids digestion and has a deflating effect. Traditionally, it is also used to relieve symptoms associated with the menstrual cycle, such as abdominal cramps and breast pain. A protective plant, wild fennel was hung above doors to protect against evil spirits in the Middle Ages. Fennel seeds placed inside locks were believed to protect the home from ghosts.

– CULINARY USES –

Fennel can be used in many dishes because of its fresh, aromatic flavor. The flowers can be used to add a touch of color to dishes, and the leaves can be added to soups. Chopped wild fennel can be added to raw or cooked vegetables for extra flavor. And minced wild fennel can be used as a seasoning to enhance side dishes, roasted potatoes, grilled vegetables, hummus, or other vegetable-based preparations. You can make an excellent pesto from the leaves, blending them with garlic, pine nuts, or almonds, along with lemon juice and salt. Add it to summer pastas, or spread it on a piece of toast.

Risotto with Wild Fennel and Lemon

YOU WILL NEED:

- 1 cup of Arborio rice (or other type of risotto rice)
- 1 diced onion
- 2 cups of vegetable broth
- 1/2 cup of dry white wine
- 1 bunch of wild fennel, leaves and stems separated and finely chopped
- Zest of 1 organic lemon
- Juice of 1 lemon
- Extra virgin olive oil
- Salt and pepper to taste

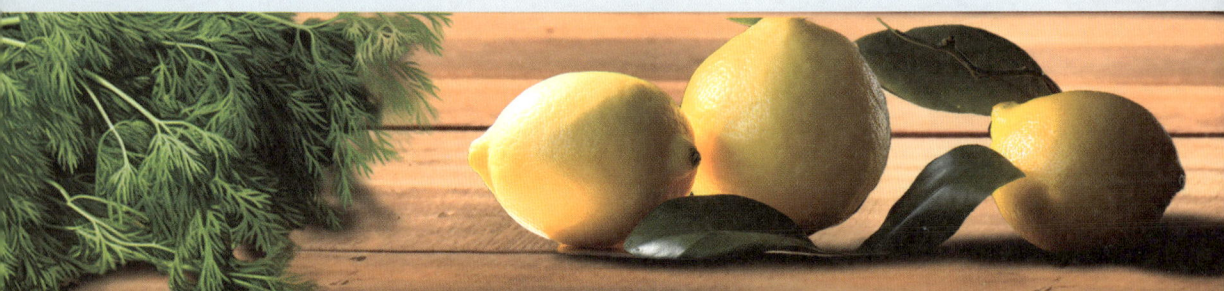

In a saucepan, heat some olive oil and add the chopped onion. Sauté it over medium heat until it becomes translucent. Add the rice, and toast for one to two minutes, stirring constantly. Pour in the white wine and let it evaporate for a few minutes, then add the vegetable broth, continuing to stir. After about ten minutes of cooking, add the chopped wild fennel and continue adding vegetable broth until the rice is *al dente* and has reached the desired creamy consistency. Adjust the salt and pepper, turn off the heat, and add the zest and lemon juice to the risotto. Stir well. Leave covered for a few minutes, then serve with a few fennel leaves for garnish.

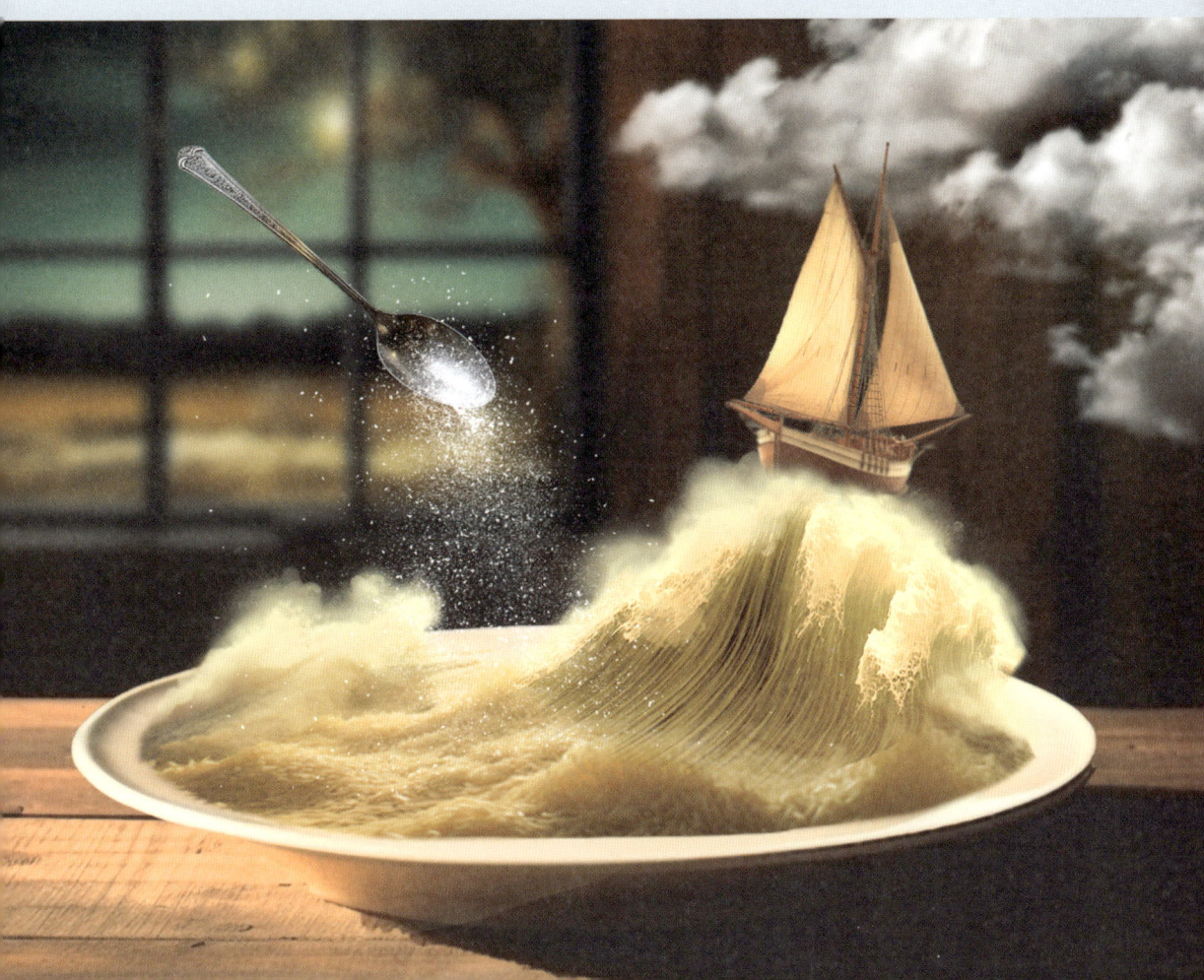

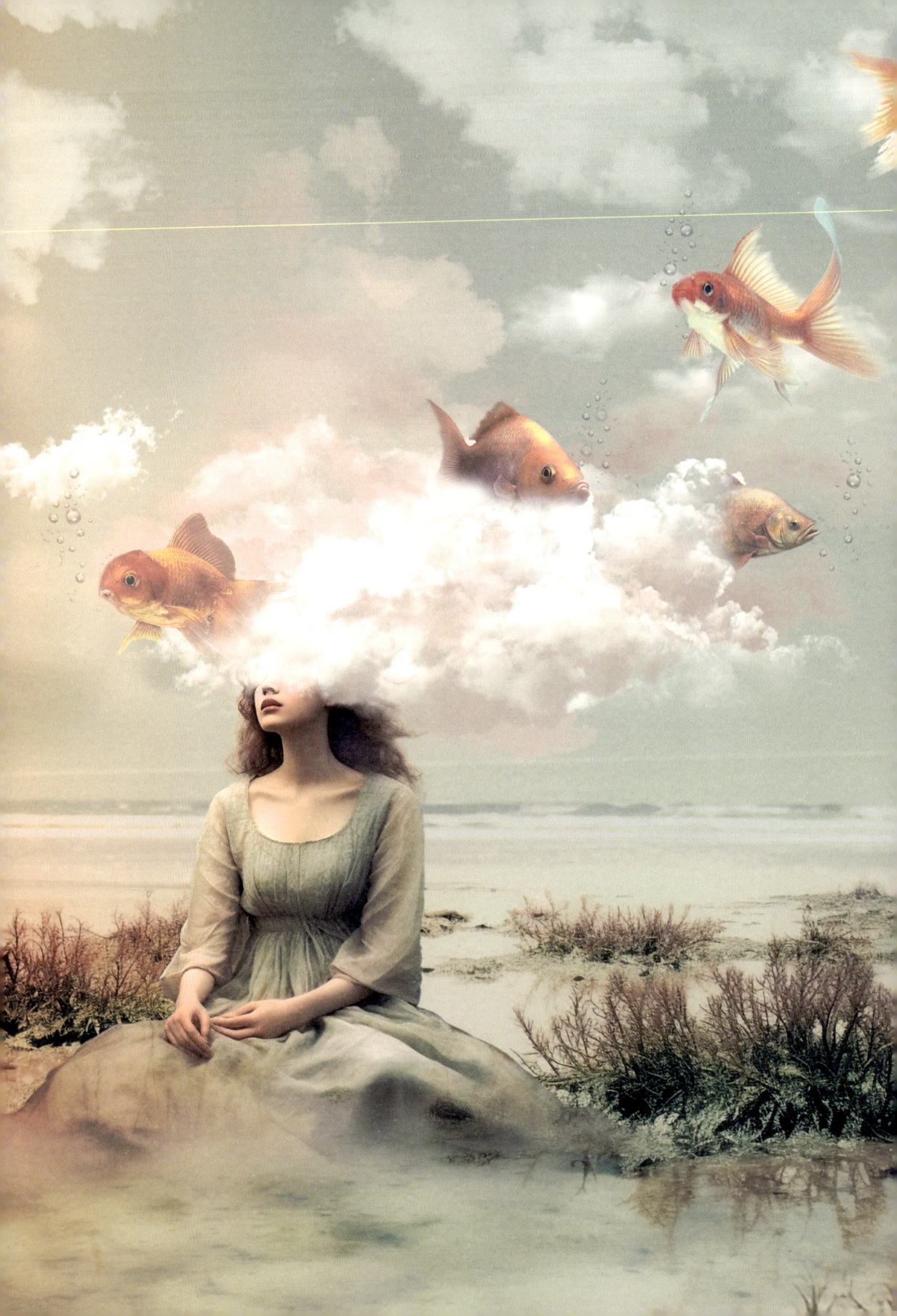

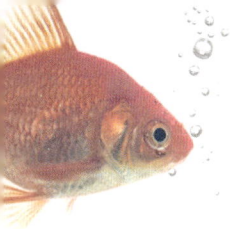

SALICORNIA

– SALICORNIA EUROPAEA –

Salicornia is a succulent plant that grows in saline soils. It possesses a large amount of protein, fiber, and minerals, and boasts of many beneficial, diuretic, and detoxifying properties. Because of its intense flavor, it is the perfect ingredient for many recipes, especially with fish and shellfish. Before using salicornia, soak it in water for at least six to eight hours to clean and remove all the salt. It is mainly found on the shoreline where the tidewater pools, and it also spreads easily in salt marshes with muddy or sandy soils. It grows in small bushes reaching a maximum height of 15 inches (40 cm). The stems are erect, fleshy, and branched, with leaves resembling small succulent scales. Rich in minerals high in protein, it is an excellent summer food. Due to its high salt content, from a magical point of view, it is a plant of protection, driving away negativity and bearing good luck.

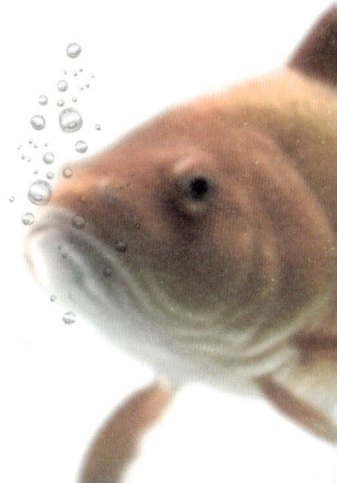

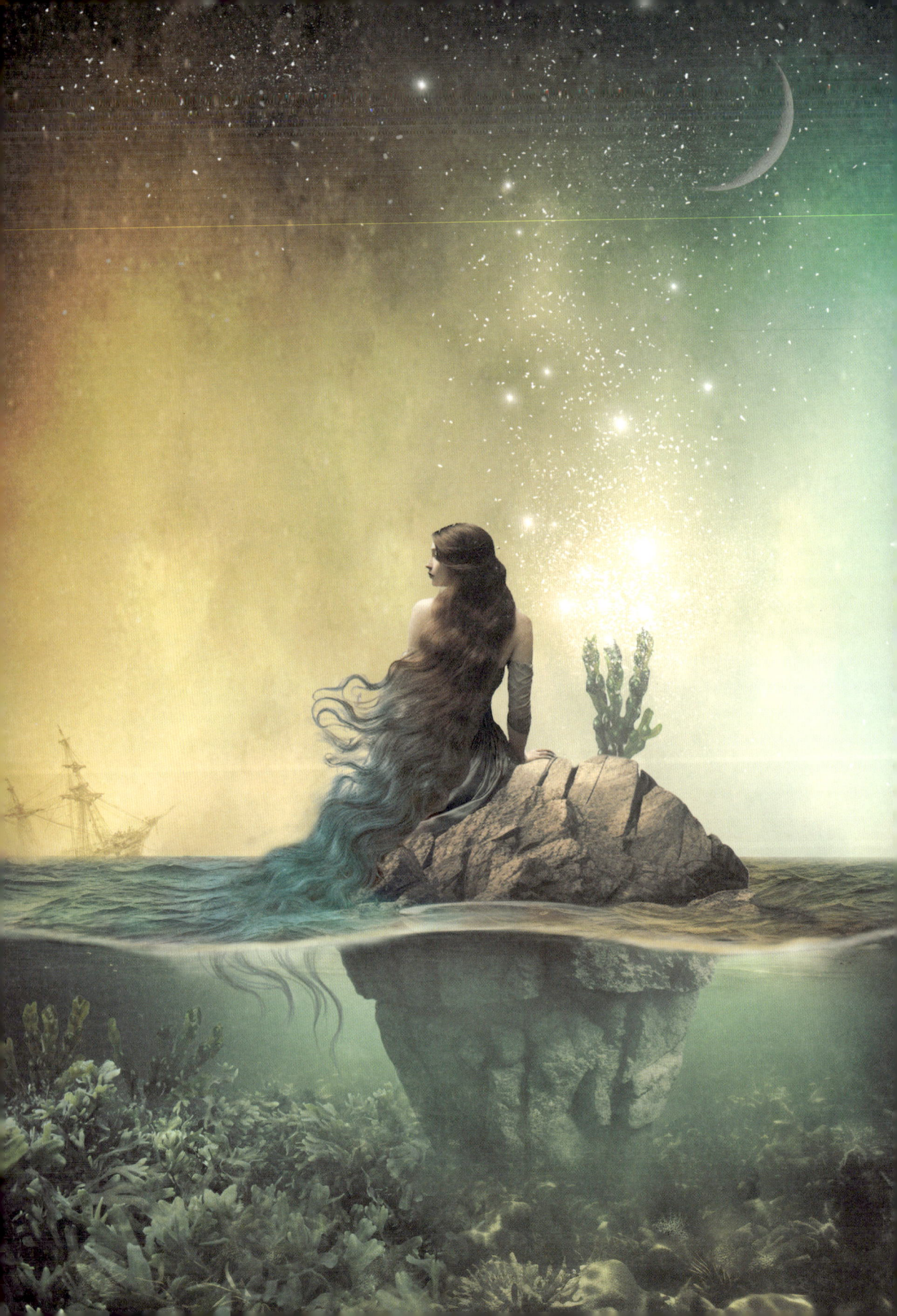

BLADDER WRACK

– FUCUS VESICULOSUS –

Bladder wrack, a seaweed known for its metabolism-activating properties, is also called sea oak. Its shape resembles that of an oak leaf. It can be used to dye things red, which is why in ancient times it was believed to be good for the blood. It is commonly found along the coasts of the Atlantic Ocean and the North Sea. It is used for its thyroid action, as it contains a lot of iodine and micronutrients necessary for the production of thyroid hormones, which are essential for increasing basic metabolism, accelerating metabolic replacement, and balancing the fat synthesis process. Therefore, the plant's stimulating action is useful in cases of hypothyroidism, but it should be taken under medical supervision if you are already taking thyroid medication. From a magical point of view, bladder wrack can be associated with problem-solving, as it brings speed of action and the ability to find original solutions.

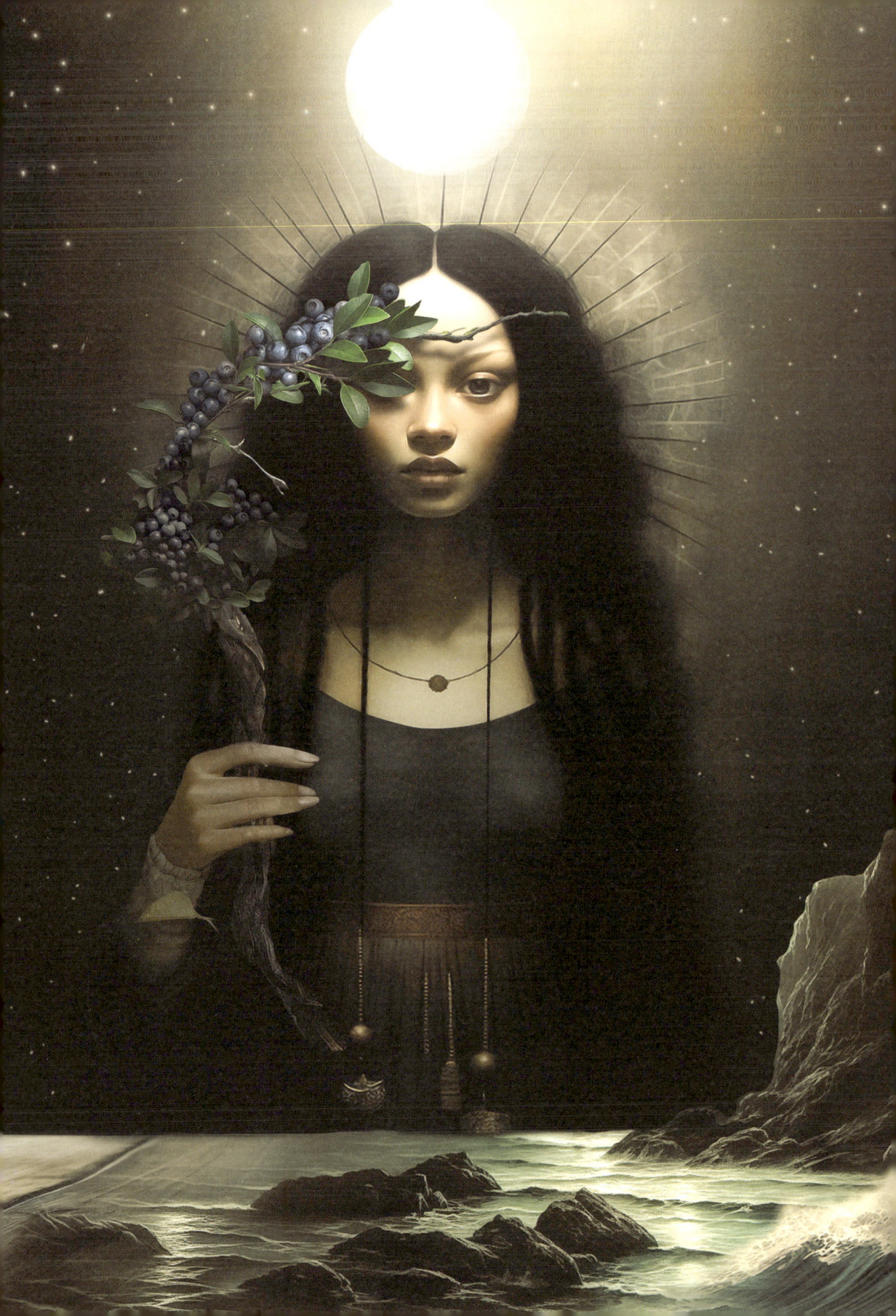

MYRTLE

– Myrtus communis –

A magical plant dedicated to Venus, myrtle is a wild plant that can be found near the sea in Mediterranean areas. It has oval, slightly elongated leaves of a beautiful, shiny dark-green color. But the real distinguishing mark of the plant is its berries, which are small and pearl-shaped. They are very fragrant and give off an intense aroma, reminiscent of eucalyptus and lemon. It has digestive properties, famous for a liquor made with the berries and consumed at the end of a meal, as well as antioxidant and antibacterial properties. It can be used to treat infections of the skin and respiratory tract, such as coughs, colds, and sinus infections. It is also used in cosmetics, to treat delicate or acne-prone skin. From a magical point of view, the plant symbolizes love, beauty, and fertility, and its flowers, which resemble the stars over the sea in summer, were often used in love rituals.

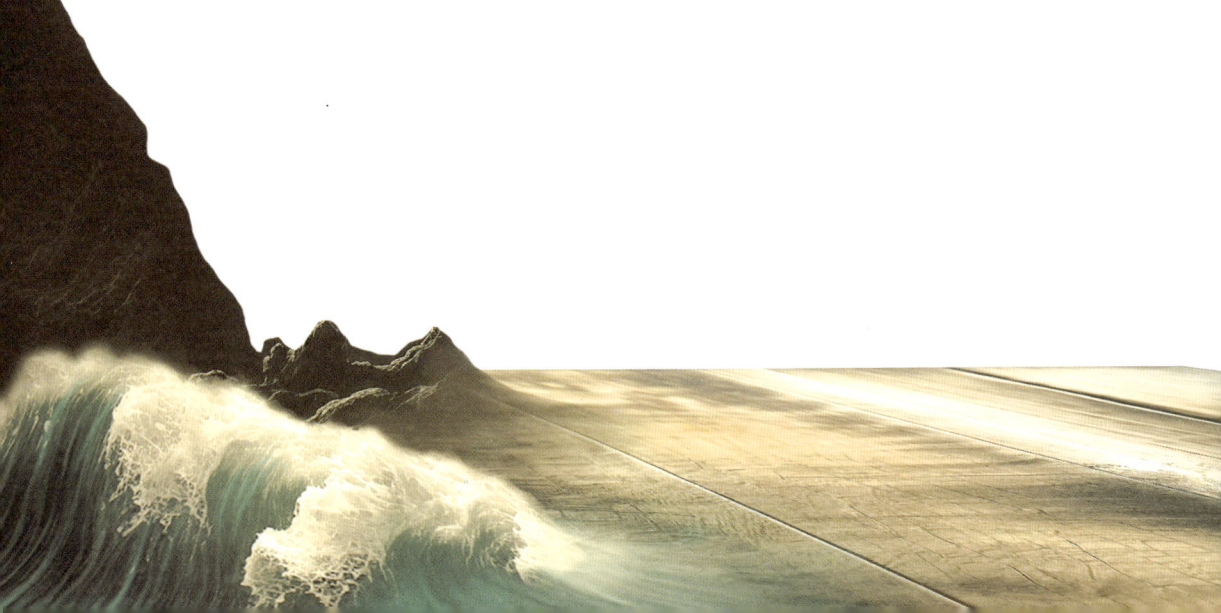

– MAGICAL USES –

Myrtle can be used in magical practices to attract love, protection, and prosperity. To create a love spell, you can gather a few fresh myrtle leaves and place them under your pillow or inside a small cloth bag. This simple gesture is believed to attract love or rekindle an existing relationship. Or you can create a talisman or amulet out of woven myrtle twigs. Hang this powerful symbol of protection on your front door. Or wear it as jewelry to create an energy shield around you, warding off negative energy and letting only the right people into your life.

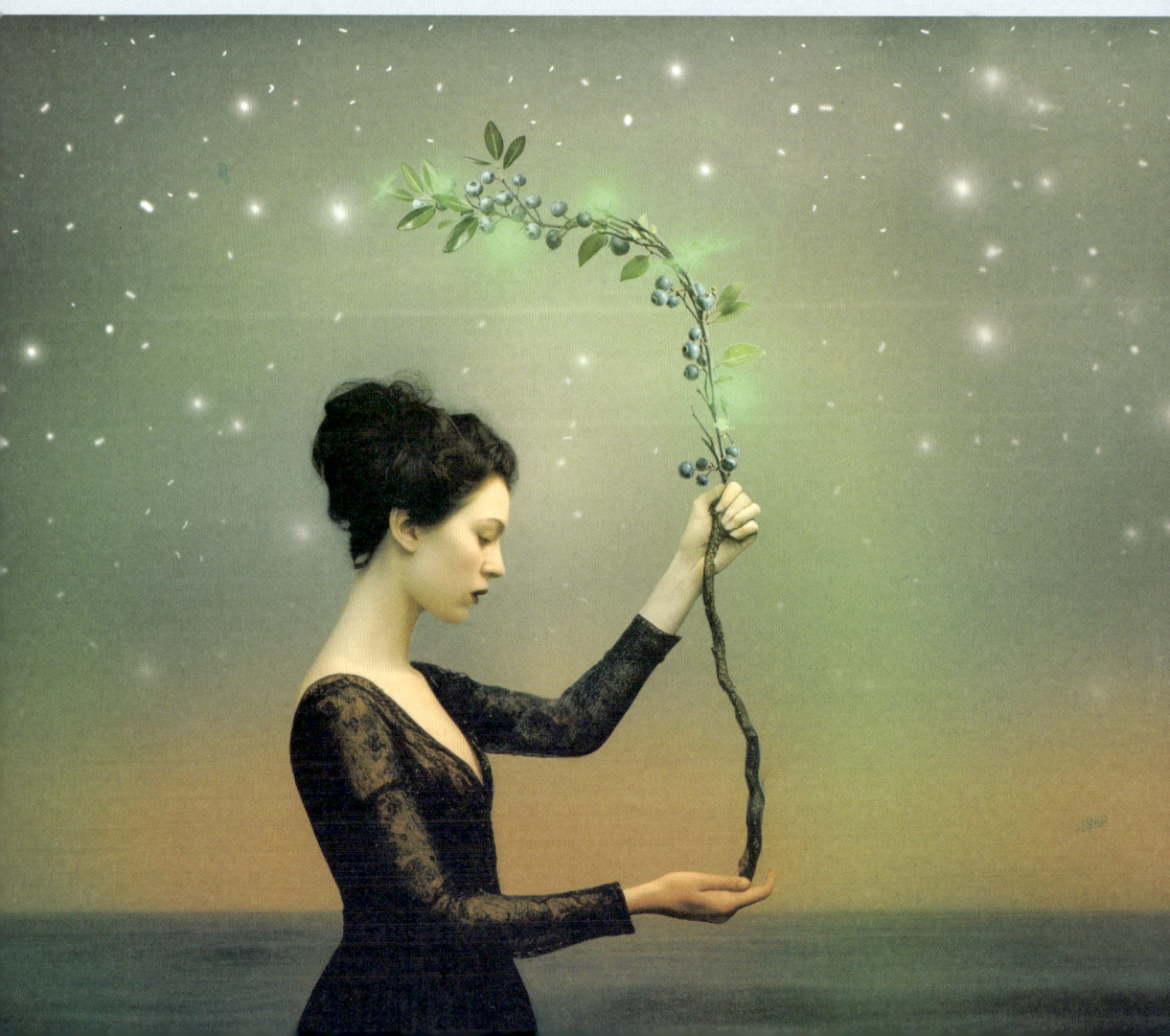

Like a Summer Star: A Ritual with Myrtle

Find a quiet, private place where you can concentrate without distraction. Gather some fresh myrtle twigs and create a sacred space by lighting a candle or placing a crystal or an object that's dear to you in front of you. Breathe deeply, take the myrtle twigs in your hands, and focus your intention on what you wish to attract into your life, be it love, protection, or any other form of positive energy. Repeat a prayer or affirmation that resonates with you, such as: *By the power of myrtle, I attract love and protection into my life. Let it be so!* Imagine a glowing green light expanding around you, surrounding the myrtle in your hands. Visualize this green light spreading into your surroundings, creating an energy field of love and protection. Now that the myrtle has been blessed and charged with positive energy, you can use it in any way you like: you can create a wreath, hang the twigs on the door of your home, or even create a wand or a small plant sculpture.

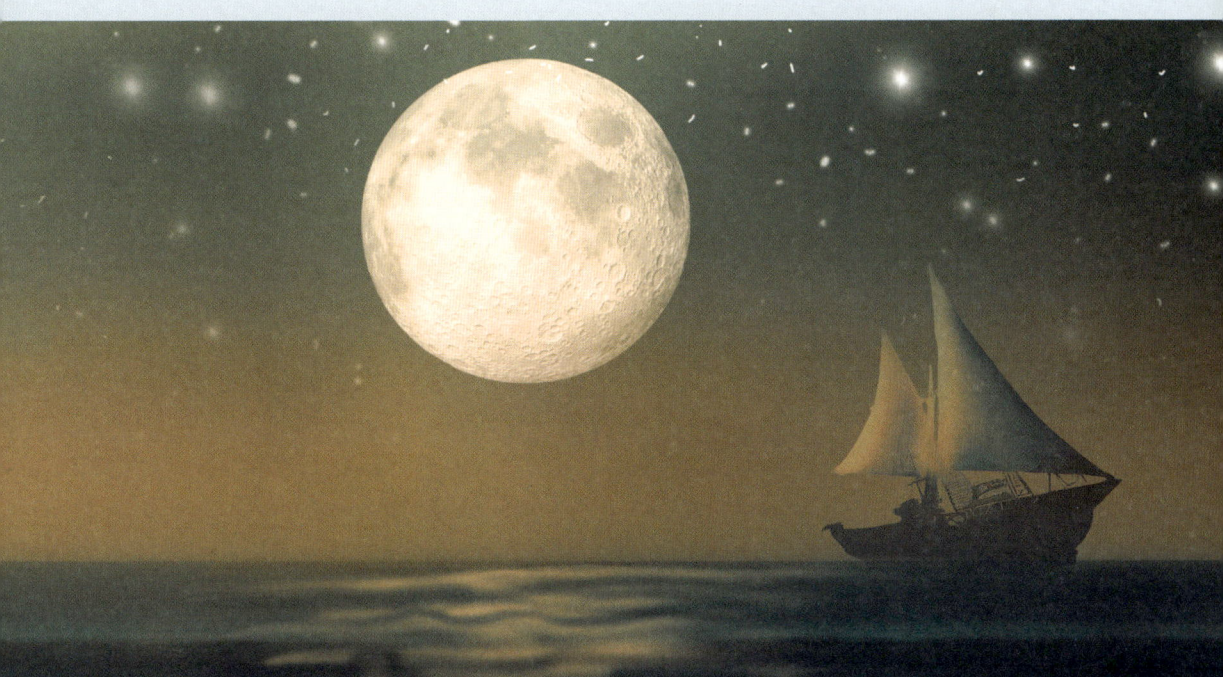

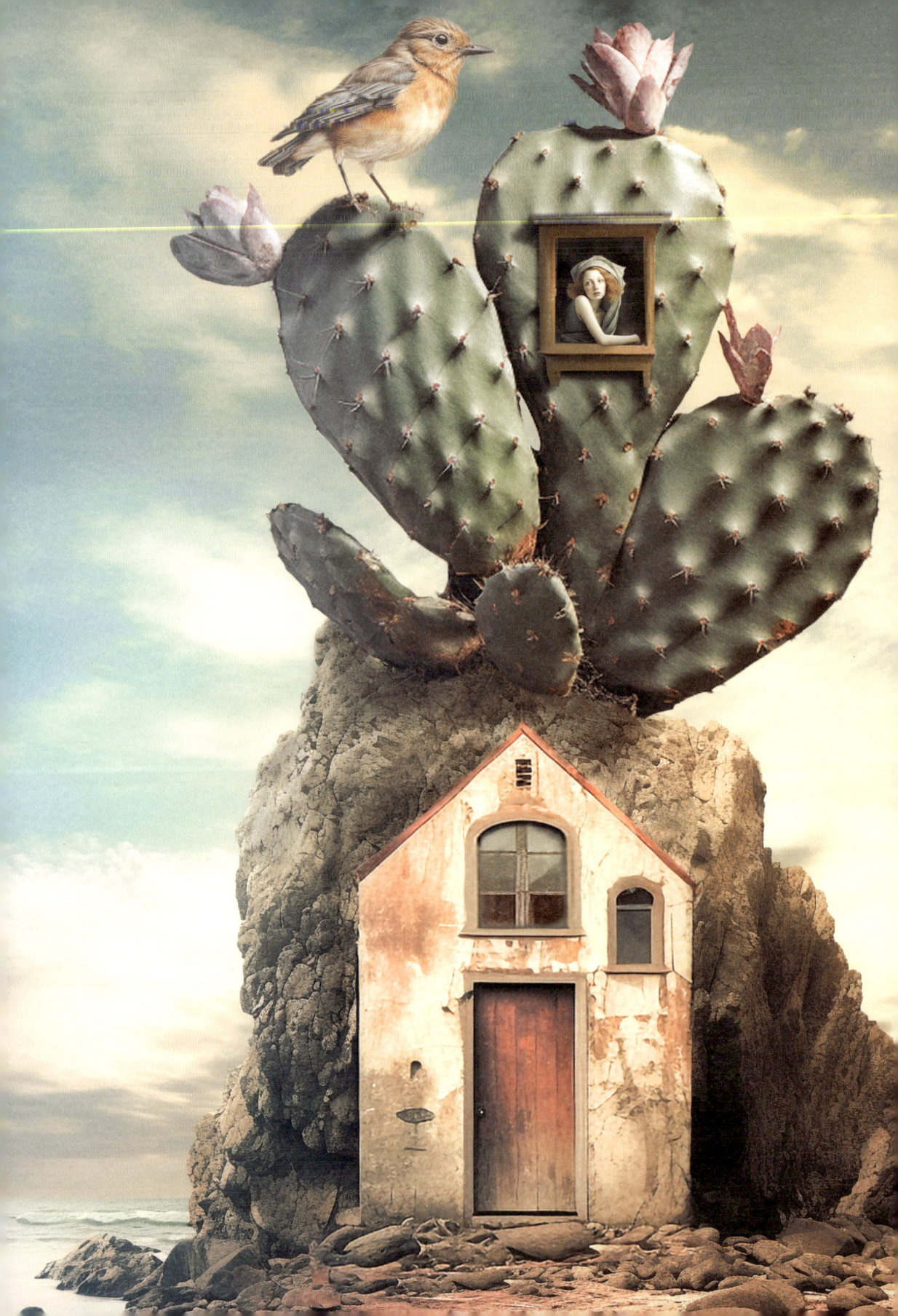

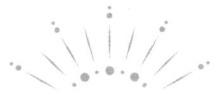

PRICKLY PEAR

– Opuntia ficus-indica –

The prickly pear is a peculiar and very recognizable plant: it can grow up to 16 feet (4.8 meters) high and has no true leaves. Instead, it has thick, fleshy, oblong, green cladodes that carry out chlorophyll photosynthesis in the place of true leaves, which have turned into sharp conical spines of about half an inch. It is a very creative plant and knows how to adapt to the driest climates. Its flowering bears fleshy fruits, which contain sweet pulp rich in minerals such as calcium, phosphorus, and vitamin C and are picked and eaten or used to prepare jellies, juices, liqueurs, and syrups. It has antioxidant effects and diuretic, healing, and soothing properties and can help reduce the symptoms of alcohol intoxication. From a subtle and magical point of view, it works on adaptability and invites you to use your full potential even in difficult situations.

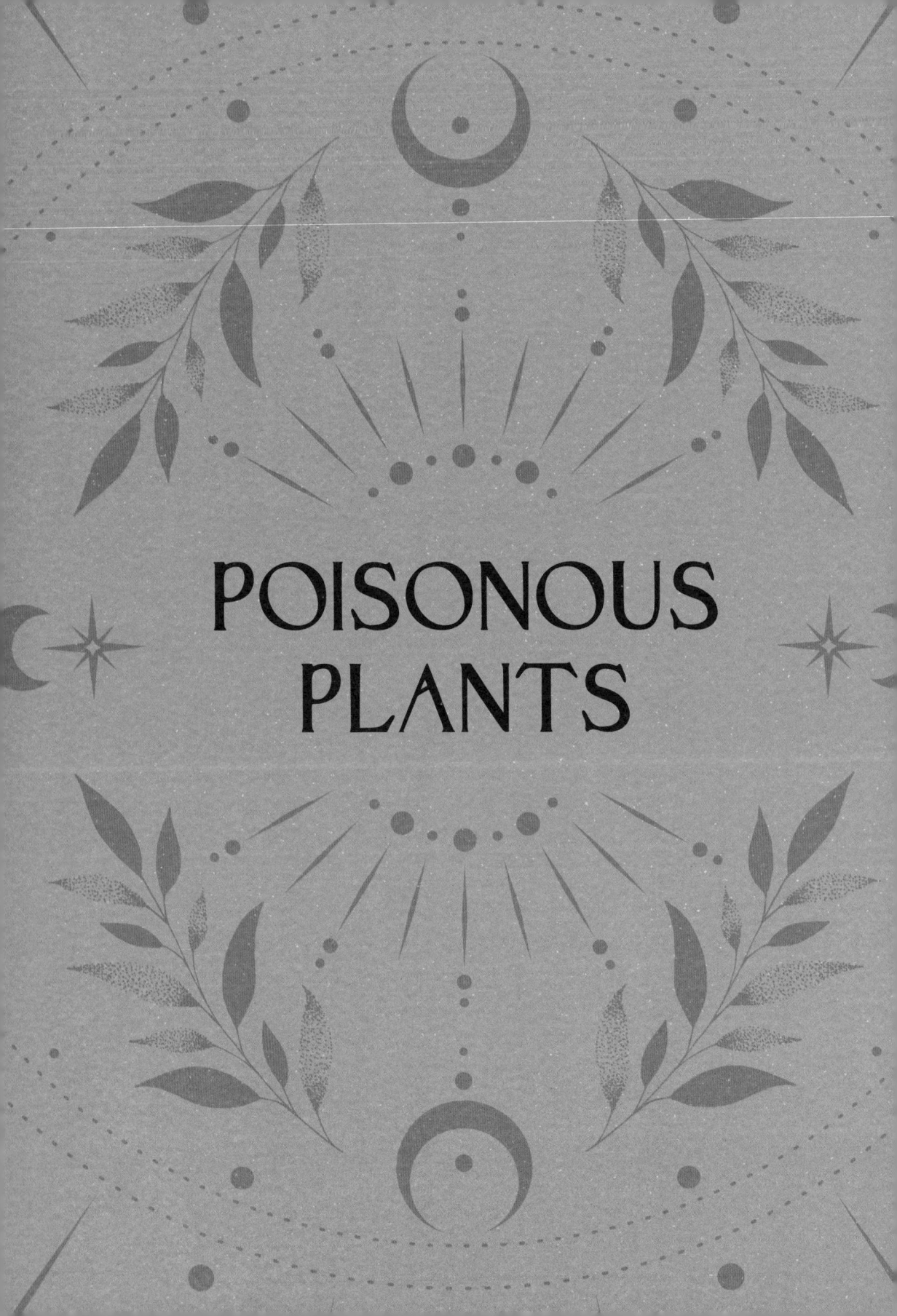

POISONOUS PLANTS

Poisonous plants have possessed an undeniable fascination forever. Their colors and the shapes of their flowers or fruits—often unusual and beautiful, like the red arils of yew or the shiny berries of nightshade—attract and intrigue. And then there are their psychoactive effects, which have made poisonous plants, although very dangerous, a constant symbol of the magical dimension and the expansion of consciousness. In ancient traditions, poisonous plants were used by shamans, witches, and magical practitioners as a means to achieve a state of trance, to travel between worlds, or to gain visions and profound insights. They are associated with power, mystery, and danger, but can also symbolize secret knowledge, transformation, and access to hidden worlds. Their duality—on the one hand dark and deadly, on the other magical and decisive—has inspired many a fairy tale in tradition, but their appeal endures today. In magical practice, they are still used, with greater regard for safety in handling them. New and more subtle ways of contacting their energy are being explored. It is important to specify that all the poisonous herbs that will be discussed in this chapter should not be ingested at all, nor otherwise used in contact with the skin or for internal use. Ointments, oils, teas, macerates, and other herbal preparations are highly discouraged. Many of these plants have powerful poisons, which can lead to extreme consequences. Approaching the world of poisonous plants means accepting the teachings of Mother Nature, learning something about limits and self-protection, and having respect and care for the plants we encounter, especially if they are as powerful and sacred as the poisonous ones.

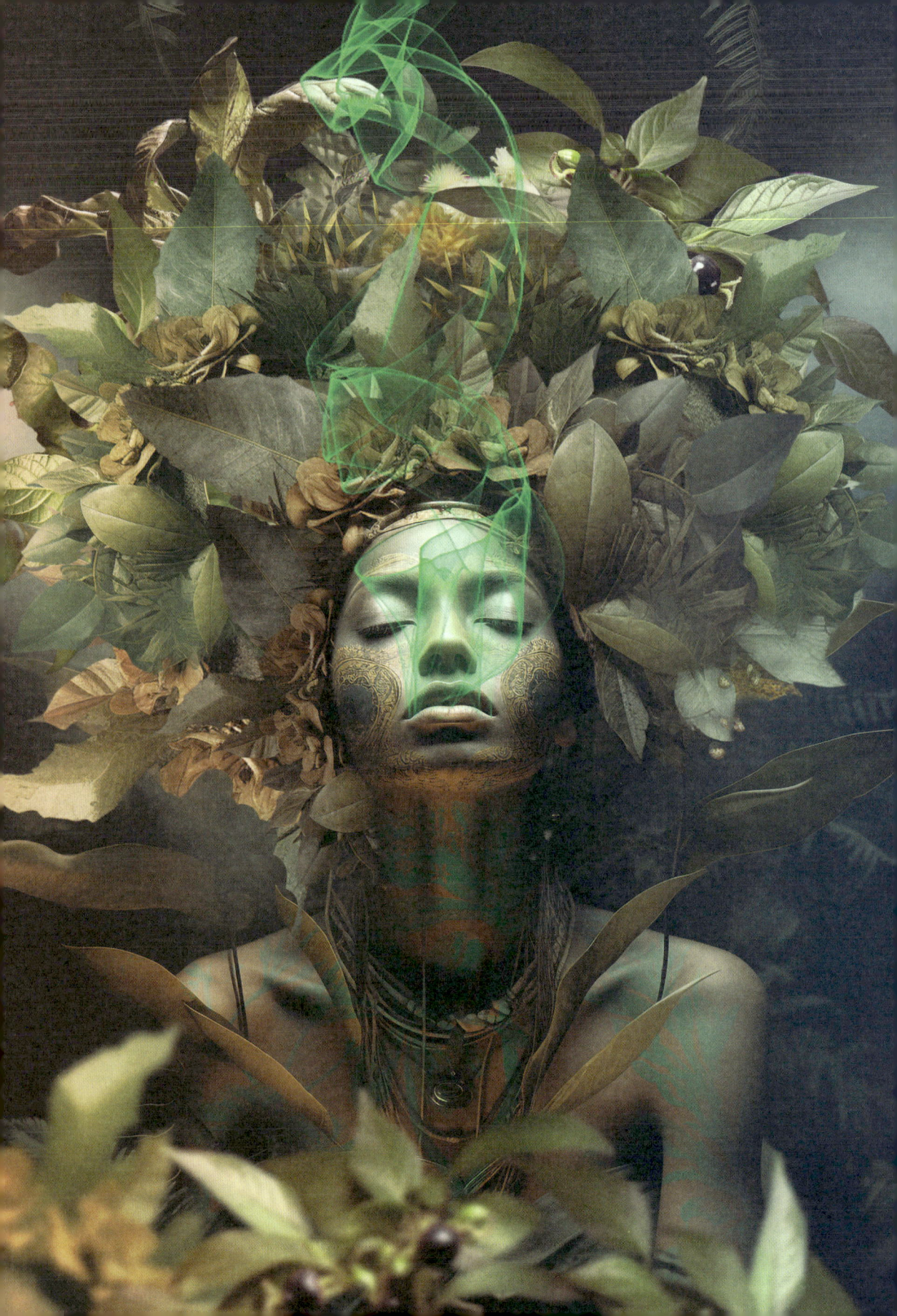

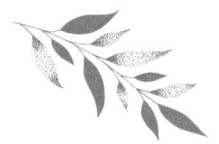

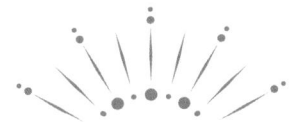

THE SHAMAN
WITCH

—

The shaman witch lives on the edge
of the forest. She inhabits the edge,
the place where the real and invisible
intertwine, where healing takes place
through stories, where storytelling
becomes real. She sews and
embroiders, listens and heals, knows
the magical way to the paths that lead
to other worlds.

She studies herbs and knows their voices, turns to them for advice and guidance, and uses them together with subtle energy to heal. She is a witch of earth and sky. She knows roots, minerals, petals, and fragrant leaves, and she knows how to travel in the spirit world and in dreams. She knows that magical power resides in each individual and in connecting with the unseen world.

She uses rituals, spells, and sacred practices to venture into the realms of the invisible, where she interacts with the spirits of nature, ancestors, and animals. She is a bridge between the visible and invisible worlds. She embraces duality and understands the interconnectedness of all things.

The shaman witch travels between worlds through shamanic journeying, which is a method of altering consciousness. In this way, she is able to communicate with spirits, receive visions or messages, and gain profound knowledge. She uses specific techniques to go on a journey and achieve an altered state of consciousness: drumming, dancing, rhythmic breathing, chanting, or the use of sacred plant substances.

Through the practice of journeying, she seeks to bring balance, harmony, and healing to herself and to the community around her.

She works for the collective good, seeking to heal the wounds of the soul and restore the balance between humans and nature. That is why she lives on the edge, where every initiatory rite was performed in ancient times. The rites of passage of the seasons and the various ages of life were celebrated here, festivals in which the natural cycles and transitions of the seasons are honored. The spring equinox, summer solstice, autumn equinox, and winter solstice are celebrated through rites that in some traditions are called *sabbaths*.

> During *sabbaths*, the shaman witch connects with the unique energy of each season, honoring the growth, abundance, rebirth, and reflection of nature, in harmony with it.

The same thing happens with the passages of life: adolescence, adulthood, old age, death. Here, on the edge, life and death are celebrated. The edge becomes a place of power from which it is possible to observe the center, in a global design that includes the complexity and resources of each. The shaman witch is a traveler between worlds and, at the same time, she is the witch most connected to the sense of humanity: guiding and inspiring, she shows us the path through the forest.

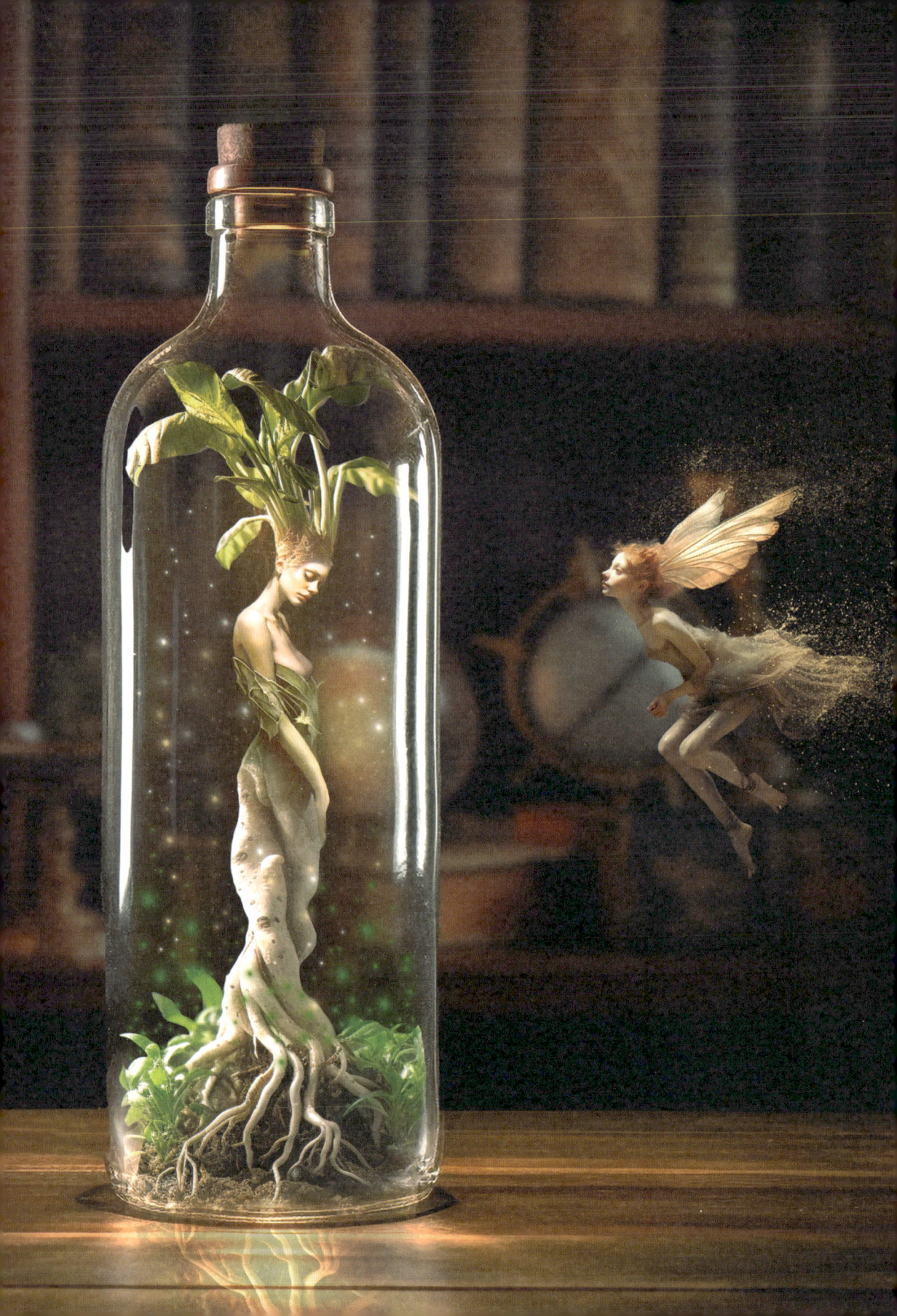

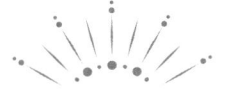

MANDRAKE

— Mandragora officinarum —

This anthropomorphic root is mentioned by Shakespeare in *Romeo and Juliet* and in the herbology lessons of the *Harry Potter* saga. Mandrake is powerful, fascinating, and very poisonous. It has large oval leaves and produces purple or white flowers. Its most distinctive feature is its large, fleshy root, which often splits into two or more branches resembling human figures. Legend has it that mandrake root cannot be pulled out of the ground; otherwise, the plant will begin to scream, which can lead to madness. Due to the shape of its root, mandrake was associated with fertility and the goddess Aphrodite. The plant was believed to be a gift from the gods and could supposedly help couples wanting to conceive simply by carrying a piece of its root. Every part is toxic, so its use is strongly discouraged.

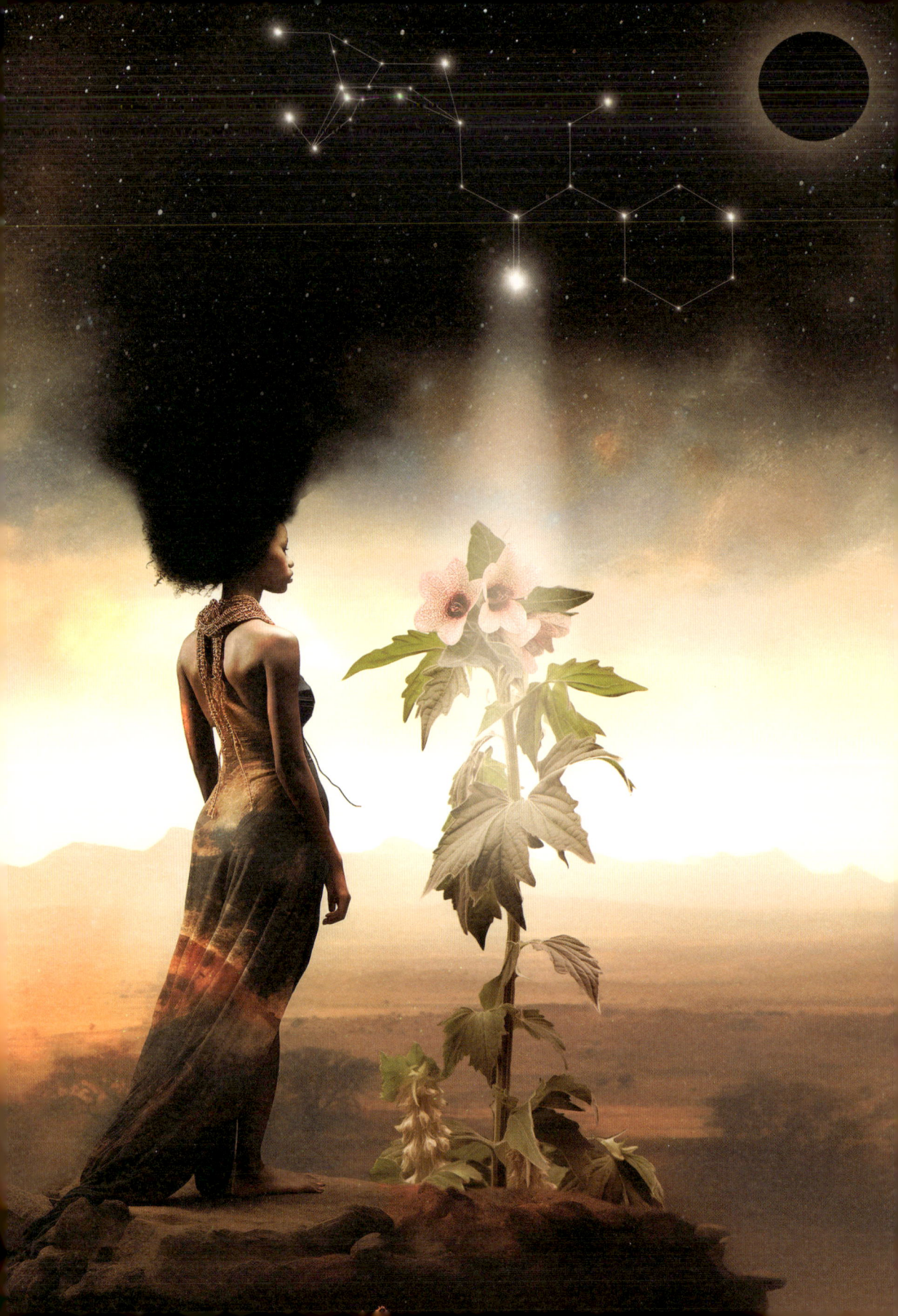

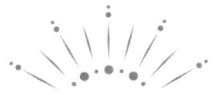

HENBANE

— Hyoscyamus niger —

Henbane belongs to the Solanaceae, the same family as tobacco, mandrake, nightshade, peppers, and potatoes. It blooms in late summer and has yellow flowers with purple veins. It produces pyxis-shaped fruits, which are capsules containing bean-shaped brown seeds. The plant gives off an intense and distinctive odor, which can be described as a combination of sweet and sour. Henbane has been used in the past for magical and spiritual purposes. Due to the alkaloids in the plant, it was used to induce visions and trance states in shamanic practices; the alkaloids act on the central nervous system and can cause hallucinations and delirium. Like other psychoactive plants and fungi, henbane was used for divinatory, magical, and religious practices; therefore, the plant is linked to the ability to see beyond, imagine, and develop visions of the future.

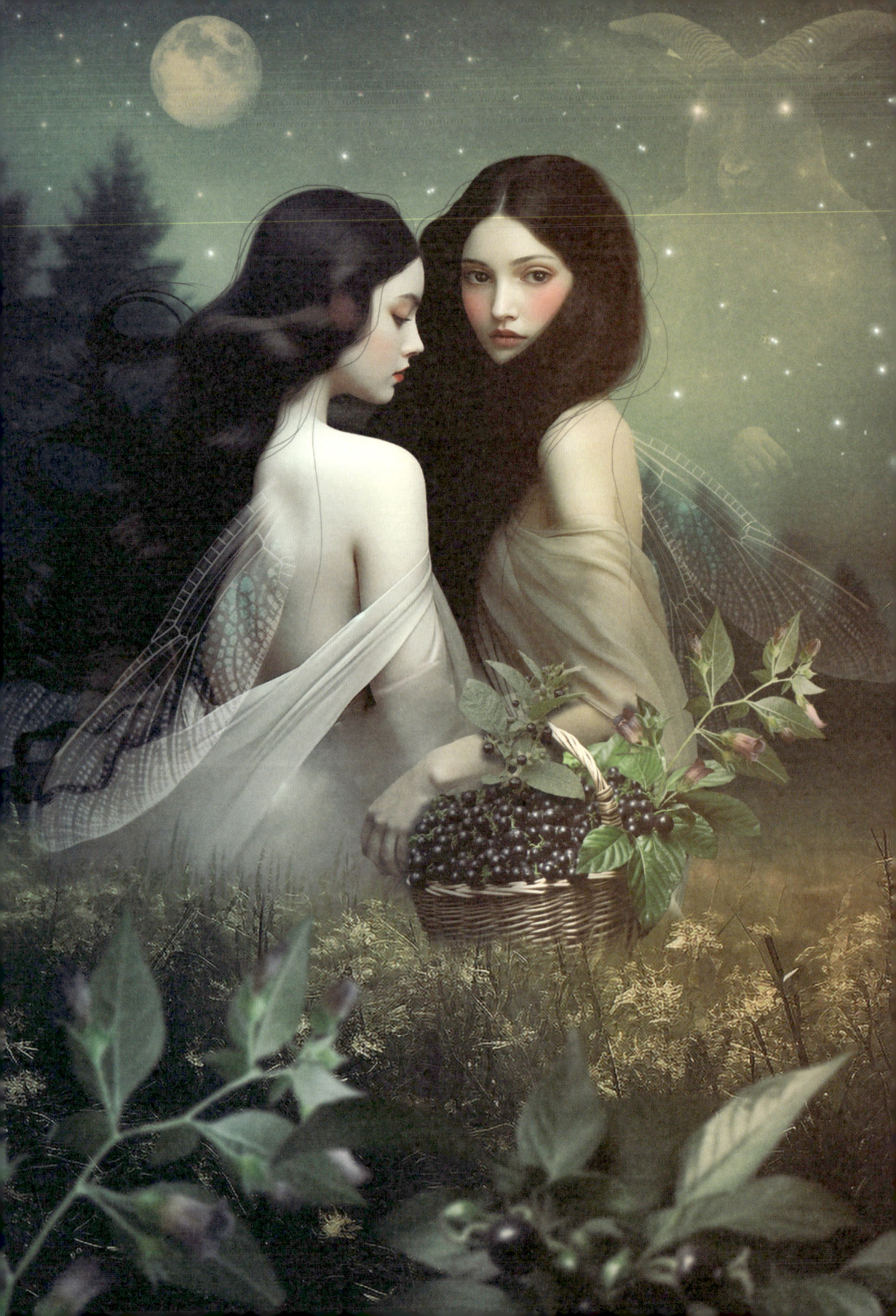

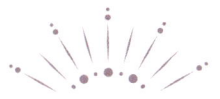

BELLADONNA

– ATROPA BELLADONNA –

Its name *Atropa* refers to Atropos, one of the three mythological Parcae, or Fates, who would sever the thread of life, a clear reference to the lethality of this plant. The word *belladonna*, on the other hand, derives from its mydriatic property, atropine, a substance in the plant that dilates the eyes and gives them a romantic gaze. Atropine was used as an eyewash and is still used in ophthalmology today to dilate pupils. The other alkaloids present, scopolamine and hyoscyamine, can have sedative, hallucinogenic, and toxic effects on the central nervous system. It is said that belladonna was one of the ingredients used in the witches' flying ointment, which they massaged themselves with at *sabbaths,* hence the hallucinations and sensation of flying. The plant is associated with the ability to see well, especially when we are experiencing all-consuming love. It invites us to stay anchored in reality and not blur our inner vision.

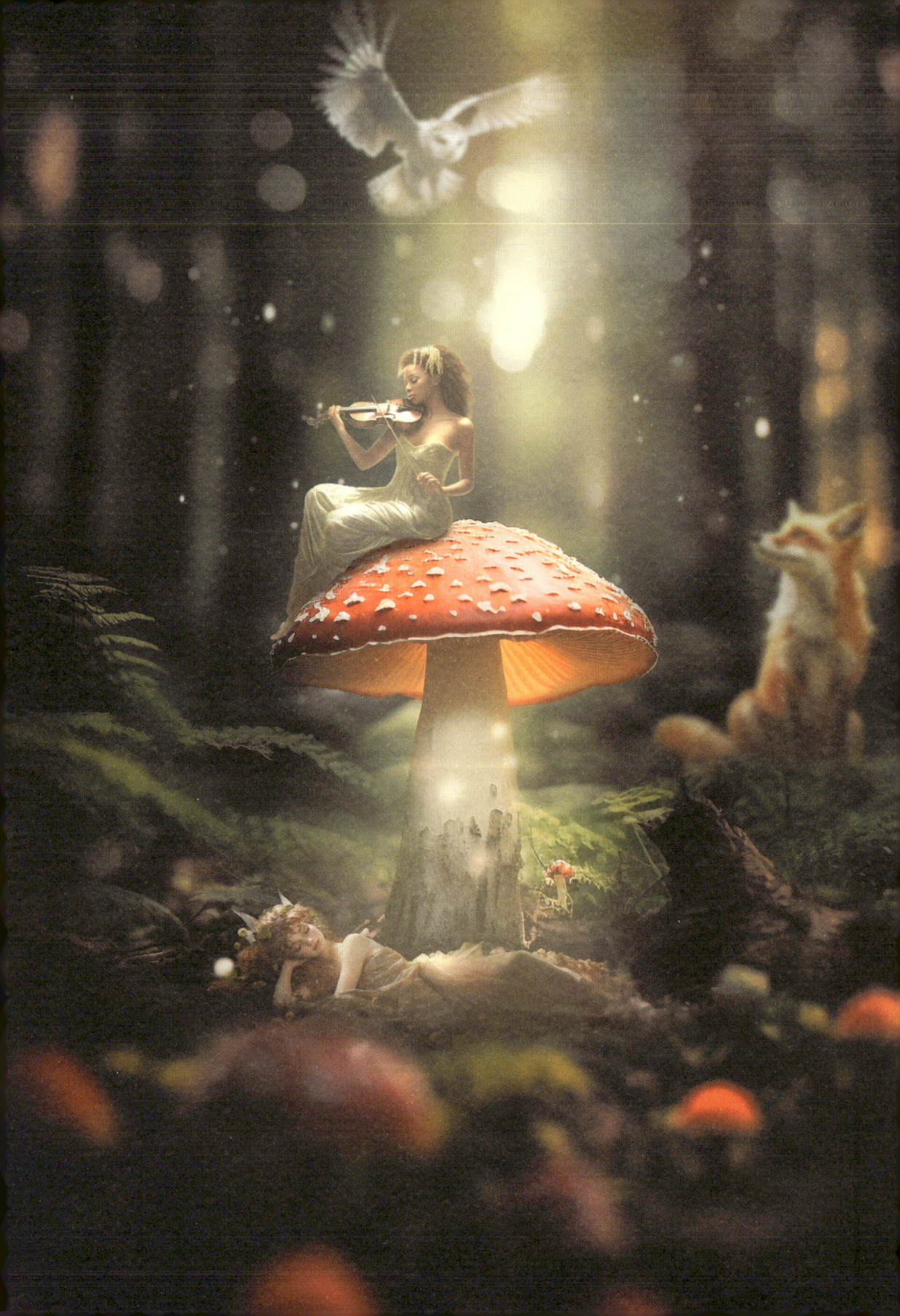

FLY AGARIC

— Amanita muscaria —

The fly agaric, with its white-dotted red cap, has become an icon in the world of magic, fantasy, and fairy tales. It is found in several shamanic traditions, particularly in Siberia. Siberian shamans consume the mushroom to alter their consciousness and facilitate contact with the spirit world. The mushroom is often consumed as an infusion, or dried and then ingested or chewed. The sensation caused by the psychoactive substances in the mushroom induces states of ecstasy, hallucinations, and connection with the spiritual world. The effects can range from a feeling of euphoria and happiness to a sense of deep connection with nature. The mushroom induces the phenomenon of macropsia, or seeing things much larger (or much smaller) than they actually are, much like what happens in Lewis Carroll's *Alice's Adventures in Wonderland*. As fly agaric is a toxic mushroom, consumption in any form is strongly discouraged.

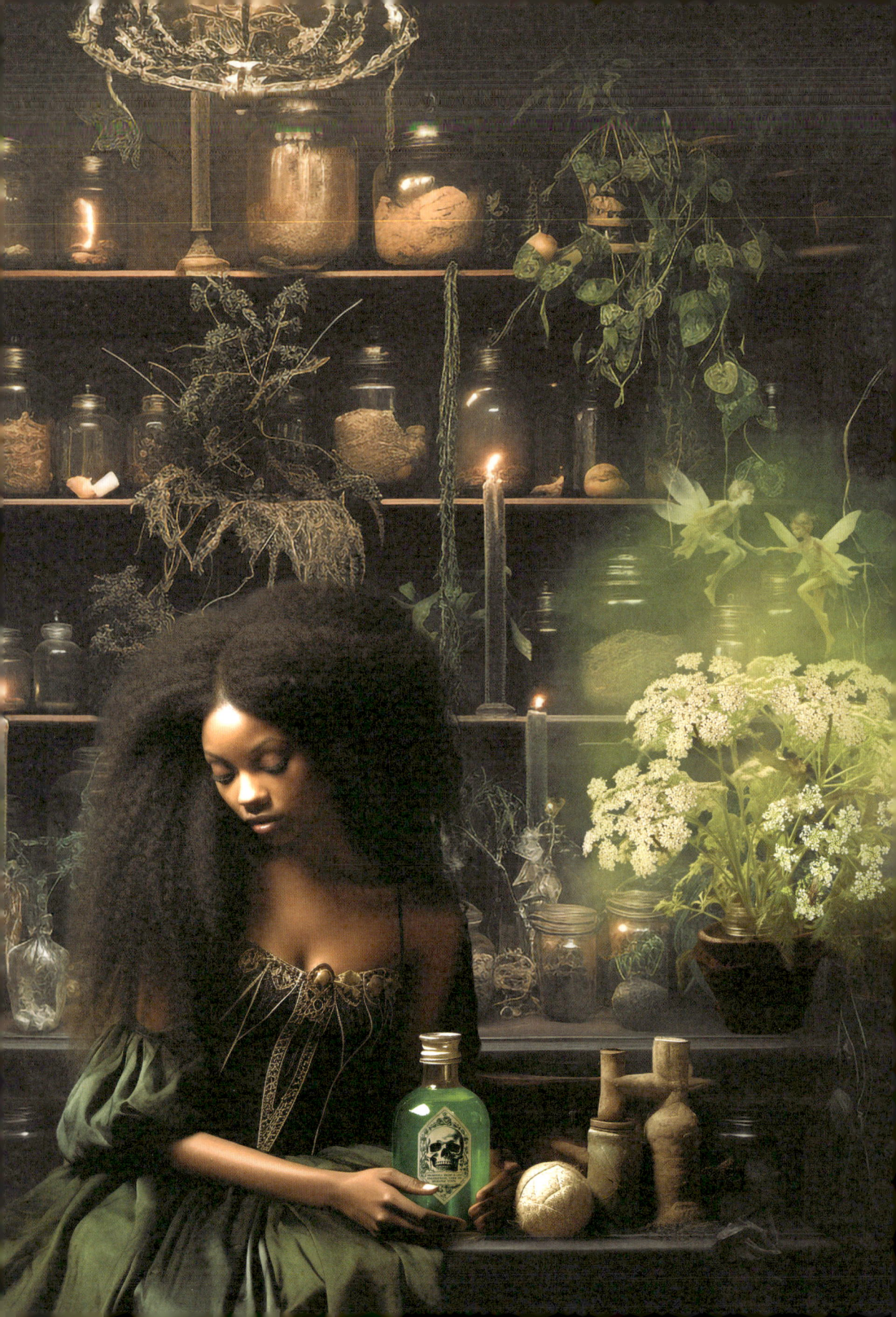

HEMLOCK

— Conium maculatum —

Hemlock belongs to the Apiaceae family, which includes common plants like parsley, dill, and cilantro. It is very important, therefore, to know how to recognize it. When collecting plants from this family, it is always advisable to have them checked by someone experienced in botany. Hemlock's stem is grooved and has purplish spots, and its smell is pungent and unpleasant. In history, the plant is closely linked to the Greek philosopher Socrates, who was sentenced to die from hemlock poisoning. His conviction was a punishment for questioning the beliefs and authority of ancient Athens. Hemlock, in this context, symbolizes oppression of authority toward free thought and freedom of expression. From a magical perspective, hemlock is often associated with the ability to reveal hidden truth or to unveil hypocrisy.

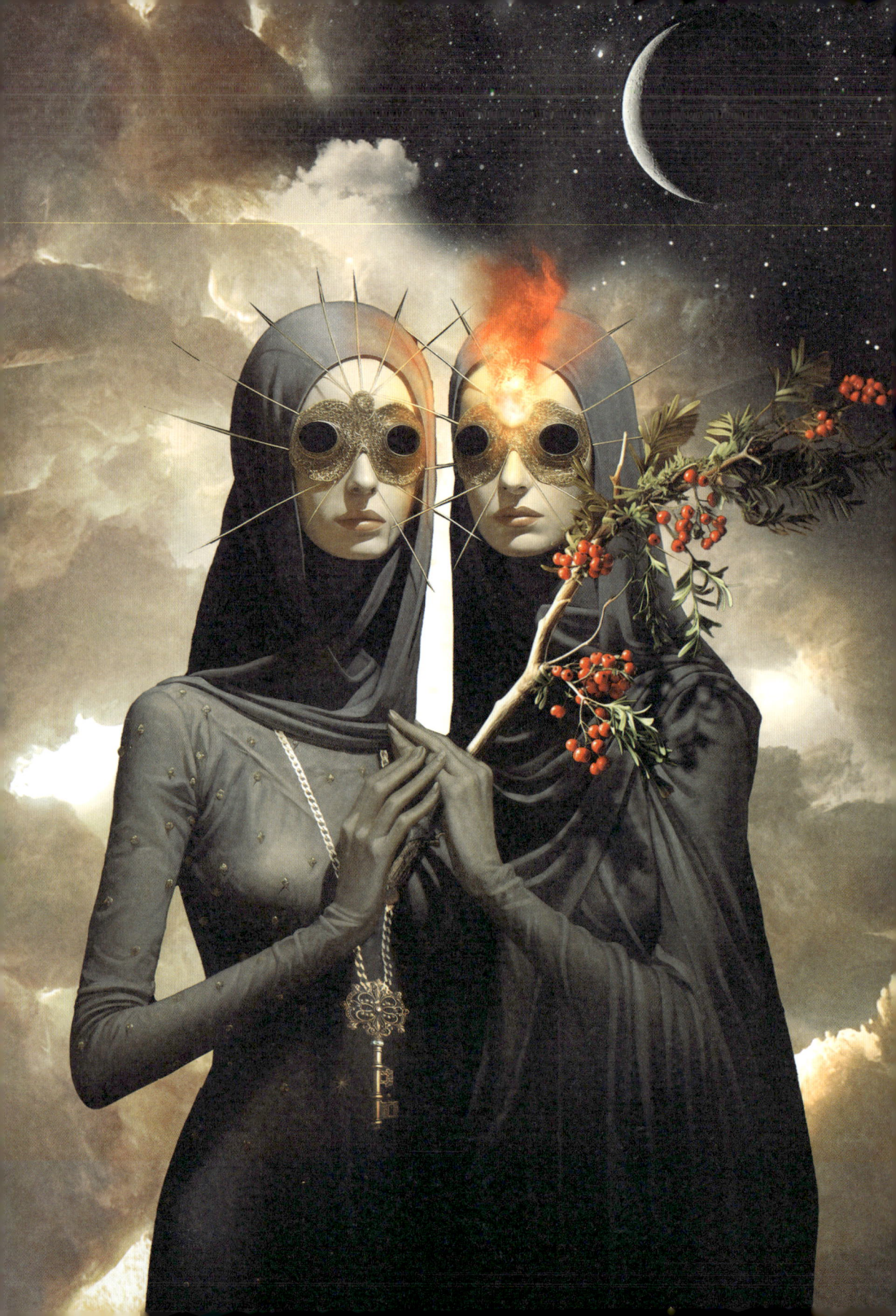

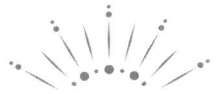

YEW

— TAXUS BACCATA —

Yew, also called the tree of death, is an evergreen that can reach great heights. It has a stout trunk, and its leaves are very dark; it produces distinctive red seeds called arils. It is mentioned by Shakespeare in *Hamlet*: yew poison poured into the ear while sleeping kills Hamlet's father. Sacred to Hecate, goddess of darkness and mystery, yew presents us with life and death as two sides of the same coin. In Eleusis, Greece, priests wore crowns of its leaves to represent death and immortality, and to symbolize the knowledge that comes from both. In Rome, on the other hand, its leaves were placed around the heads of black bulls that were offered in sacrifice to Hecate. These ancient rites unite life and death, revealing the profound wisdom that comes from accepting both. Again, given the plant's dangerous nature, caution is urged.

HOW TO ENGAGE WITH POISONOUS PLANTS

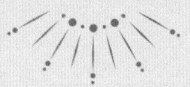

Poisonous plants are often used in magical practice, particularly in the so-called Poison Path. In magical practice, contact with poisonous herbs is based on a feeling of respect, intimacy, and awareness. The first step in exploring the "path" is accomplished through research and in-depth study of the herbs we wish to use.

> It is essential to understand their chemical properties, symbolic associations, and cultural traditions before engaging with them.

To engage with a plant, especially a poisonous plant, you can initially try using meditation. Find a quiet spot. If you are lucky enough to encounter one on a walk, you can meditate next to it. Take a few minutes to unpack your feelings, slowing down the pace of daily life. Breathe deeply and imagine the poisonous plant you want to work with.

Try to relax your mind, letting the plant open up to you and communicate its message to you. Or simply sit and listen, inhabiting the relationship between you and the chosen plant. If you want, during meditation you can ask the plant a question and then open your heart to it to receive the information and insights it can offer you. It is important to remain open and respectful, allowing the plants to guide and teach us. At the end of the meditation, you can leave an offering for the plant, whether you meditated near it or just imagined it, such as water, fresh flowers, or whatever you feel your plant desires.

Another practice that involves the relationship with poisonous plants is observation. Through simply looking, drawing, and photographing, we can gather inspiration for our day. For example, the combination of colors can suggest a palette to wear or to use in one of our work projects. Or we can be guided in artistic exploration, experimenting with various painting techniques to bring shapes and colors back to paper, even if we do not know how to draw.

> Communication with poisonous plants requires patience and openness so that their wisdom can enter our lives and enrich our magical practice.

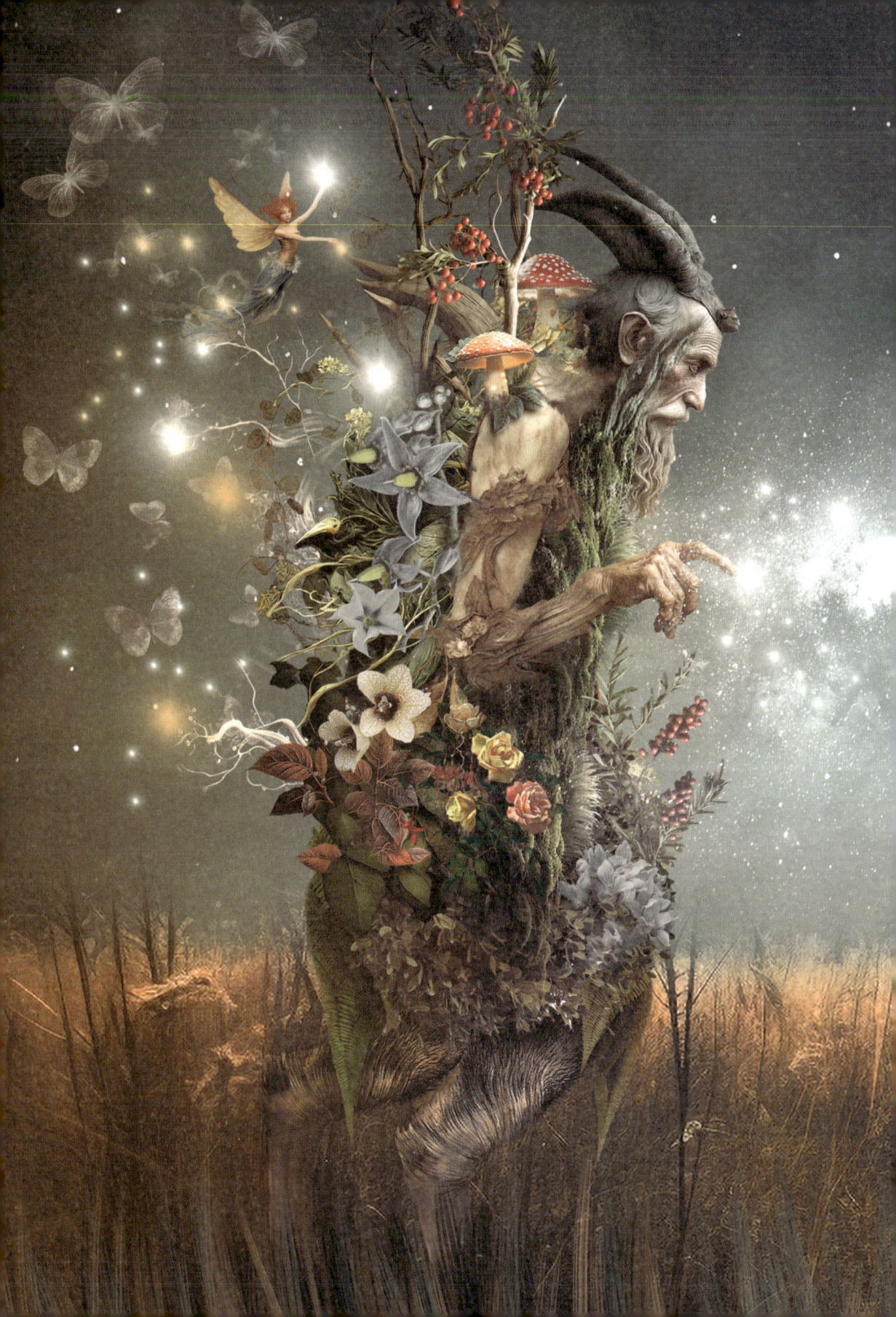

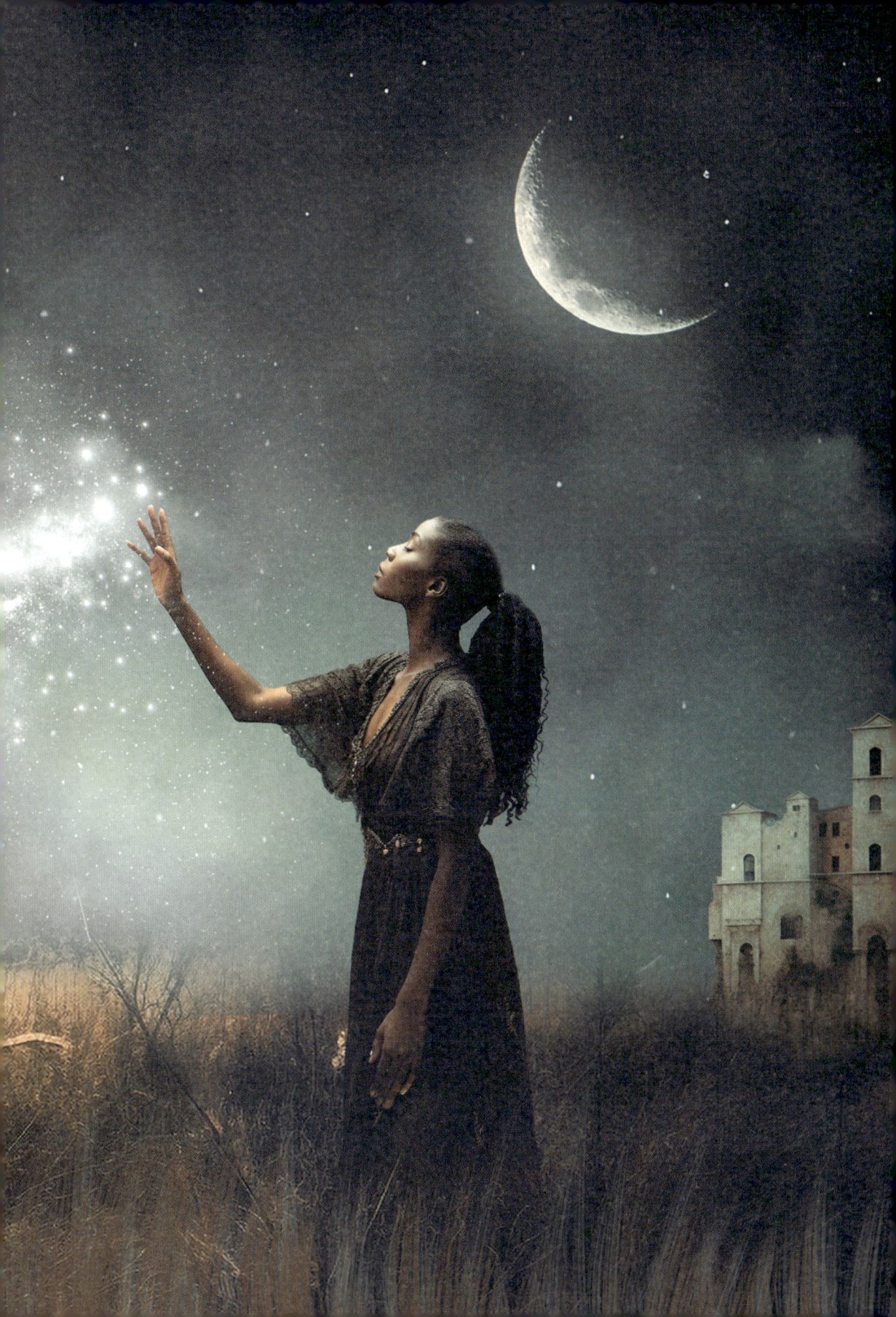

STORIES AND LEGENDS
OF THE POISON PATH

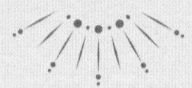

Poisonous plants, and especially the most famous
ones addressed in this chapter, evoke myths and
legends, fascinating stories that echo along the path.

Belladonna, as well as henbane, mandrake, and devil's snare, were part of the witches' flying ointment. In 1960, the director of the Institute of Ethnology at the University of Göttingen, Will-Erich Peuckert, anointed his entire body with belladonna ointment and fell into a deep sleep for 20 hours. When he awoke, he reported that he had dreams and visions the whole time that were related to the feelings recounted by those who had participated in the witches' *sabbaths*. In the countryside, people were advised against adorning themselves with belladonna flowers because it was thought to bring misfortune. At the same time, however, it was believed that planting belladonna at the beginning of the road leading home helped keep evil spirits away. Devil's snare, on the other hand, is famous for its beautiful flowers, which open only at night and have a nauseating odor. Its seeds, unlike the other parts of the plant, have a sweetish taste that is not altogether unpleasant. Courtiers and brigands in Old Europe added them to drinks to make the unwary drinker lose his will completely and start telling all his secrets. Another fascinating plant is wolfsbane, with its beautiful electric blue flower, also called devil's helmet for the shape of the petals. Its poison was used to anoint the blades of swords to make them even deadlier weapons.

According to myth, the plant originated from the slime of Cerberus, the giant three-headed dog that Hercules brought to Earth in one of his labors. It has a strong connection with wolves because its poison was used in meat patties for poisoning wolves when they got too close to houses. Wolfsbane powder was also said to keep werewolves away. It is a protected species and should not be collected, in part because it is very dangerous. Poisoning can occur from simple skin contact with the flower. Henbane was considered sacred by the Celts, particularly associated with the god Belenus: it was said that it could only be picked by a virgin, provided, however, that the virgin walked home backward. The laws of ancient Britain considered it more serious to offend the yew tree than a person, since the tree could not defend itself. In Ireland, the yew tree is believed to be the oldest of the trees created in Earthly Paradise, and the wheel of the Apocalypse of the druid Mug Ruith is made of yew wood. These are just some of the legends about poisonous plants. It is important to remember that these plants require deep knowledge and careful, responsible use.

Poisonous plants continue to enchant and fascinate as living testaments to our connection with the plant kingdom and its ability to bestow life, healing, and death.

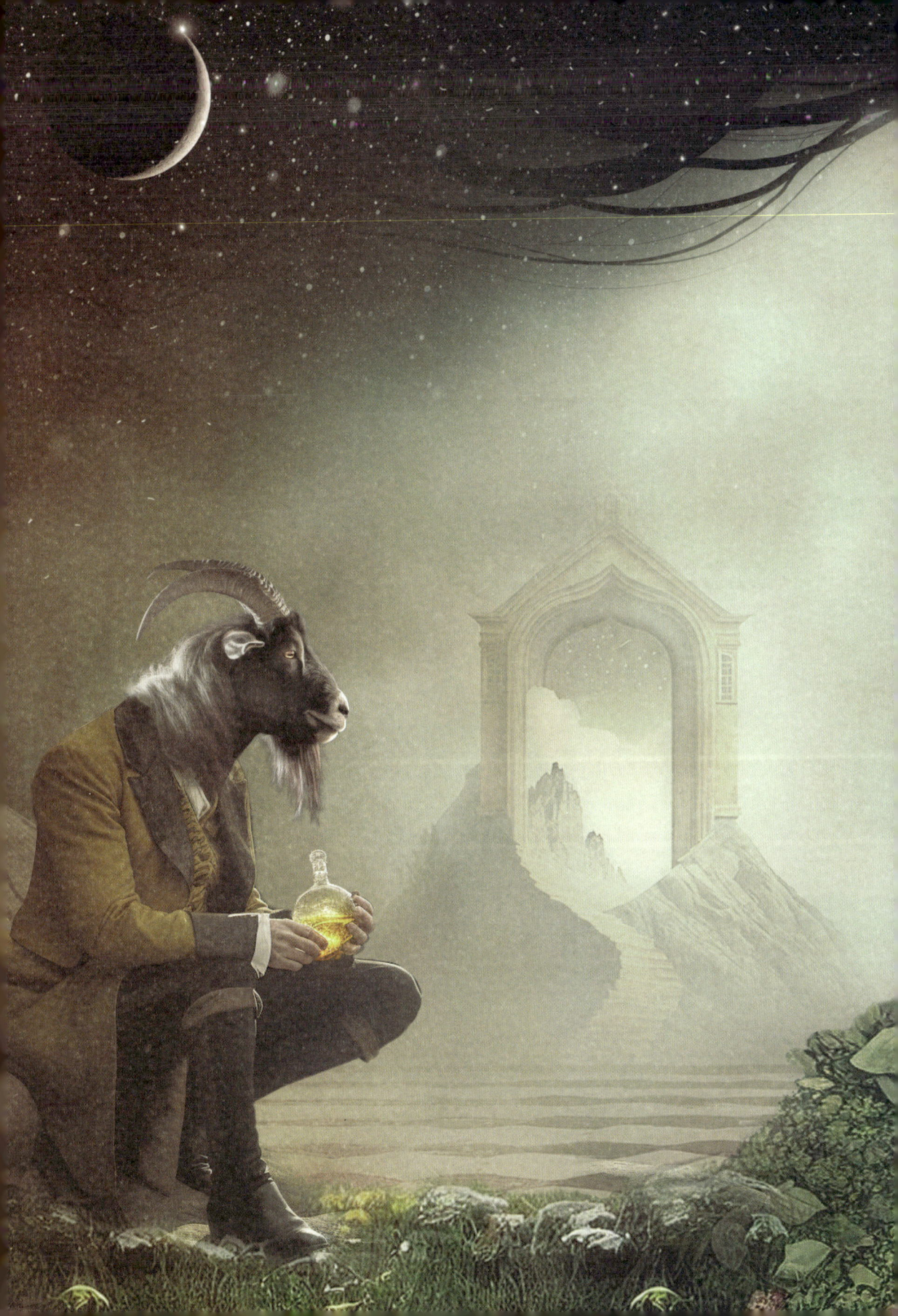

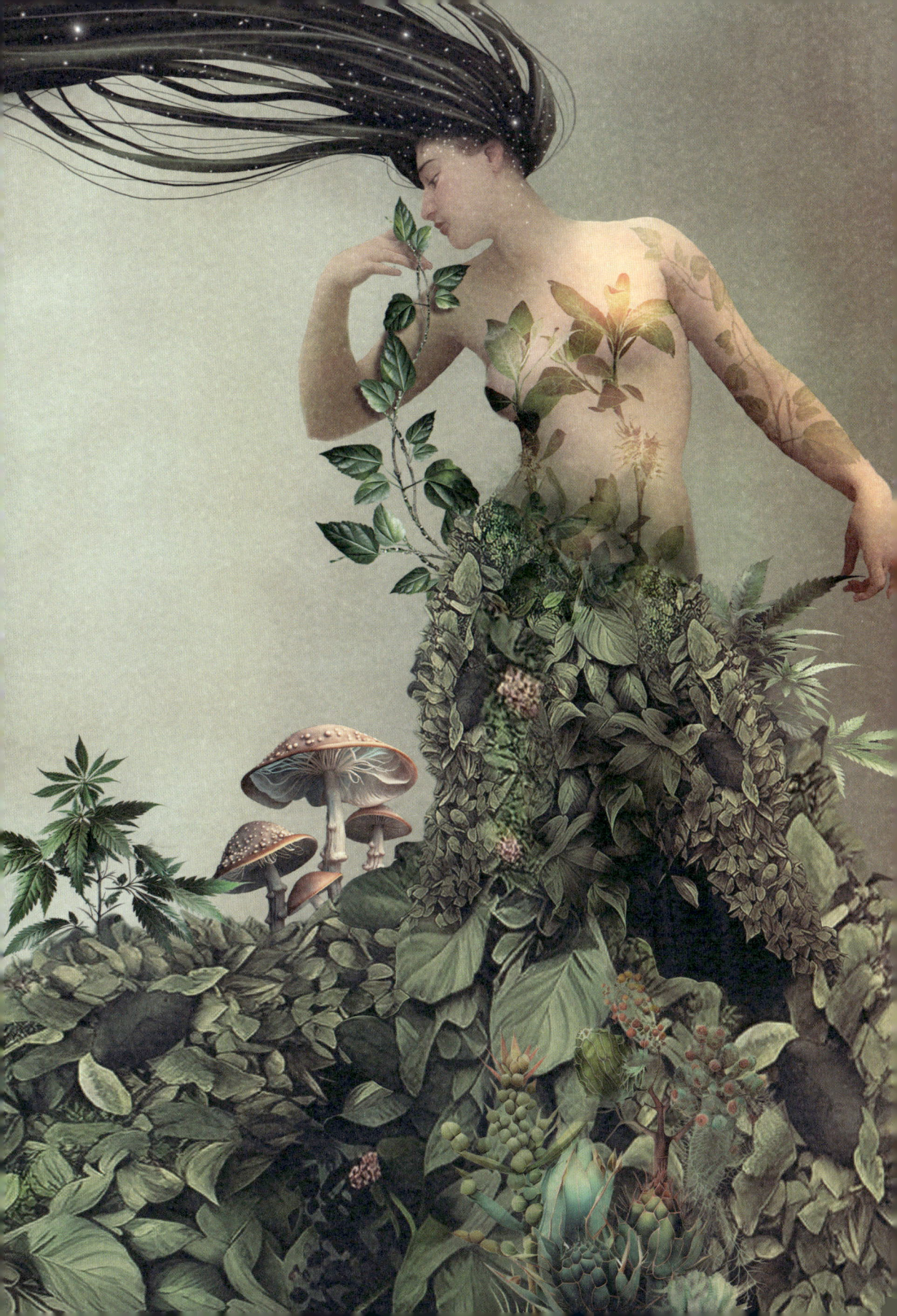

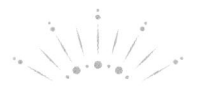

CECILIA LATTARI

Cecilia Lattari is an herbalist who studied at the University of Bologna. She is a teacher of social pedagogy who works through various media: writing, theater, contact with the natural world, and relationship support. Her published works include *Backyard Witchcraft* and the tarot deck *Rebel Witches Tarot*. She lives in a small town in the Tuscan Apennines near the woods.

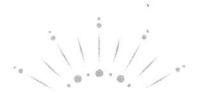

FABIANA BELMONTE

Fabiana Belmonte studied art and illustration in London and then in Spain. Since the early 2000s, she has been using Photoshop in her work, but she also experimented with traditional photography before devoting herself entirely to digital collage. She has designed numerous book covers for independent authors and won national and international competitions. Her works are distinguished by their surrealism and the inspiration they draw from nature, the feminine, and the dreamworld.

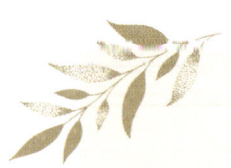

- NOTES -